Transcultural Aspects of Perinatal Health Care
A Resource Guide

Editor in Chief
Mary Ann Shah, CNM, MS, FACNM

National Perinatal Association

Library of Congress Control Number: 2002109027

ISBN: 1-58110-097-3

MA0219

Table of Contents

Contributors

John J. Botti, MD (coauthor—Professional Competence: Cultural/ Religious Efficacy and the Principles of Family-Centered Care), is professor of obstetrics and gynecology and maternal-fetal medicine at the Pennsylvania State University College of Medicine, Milton S. Hershey Medical Center in Hershey, PA. He received a bachelor of science degree from the University of Notre Dame and his medical degree from the Albany Medical College of Union University. He is a Fellow of the American College of Obstetricians and Gynecologists and a member of The Society of Maternal-Fetal Medicine. He has served and continues to serve on various state, regional, and national committees and boards and is dedicated to improving the outcome of pregnancy for families with health, educational, or socioeconomic risks.

Leonora Calsada, LCSW, MPH (coauthor—Mexican chapter), has been a clinical social worker since 1984. Her social work expertise is in perinatal settings. She is of Filipino and Mexican descent, and her specialization is on women's issues, specifically those commonly affecting women of color.

Deborah Campbell, MD, FAAP (associate editor/coauthor— Jamaican chapter), is professor of clinical pediatrics and associate professor of obstetrics, gynecology, and women's health at the Albert Einstein College of Medicine in the Bronx, NY. She is also director of the Division of Neonatology and the Low Birth Weight Infant Evaluation and Assessment Program at Montefiore Medical Center in the Bronx. Dr Campbell is a Fellow of the American Academy of Pediatrics, and board certified in pediatrics and neonatal-perinatal medicine. She has written articles, book chapters, and reviews as well as been an invited lecturer about issues relating to infant health and behavior, newborn hearing screening, and the role of families in perinatal decision making.

Sandra K. Cesario, RNC, PhD (coauthor—Jamaican chapter), is currently the director of research and an assistant professor at Texas Woman's University, College of Nursing—Houston Center where she teaches the multicultural women's health issues courses in the undergraduate and doctoral programs. Her professional career began more than 25 years ago and has focused on promoting the health of women and newborns. She was responsible for the development and coordination of the Obstetric Nurse Residency Program for the Indian Health Service. As chair of the Practice Committee and member of the board of directors for the Association for Women's Health, Obstetric and Neonatal Nurses, she plays a key role in the development of nursing practice standards in the United States and Canada. Dr Cesario's research interests include multicultural labor support practices, the use of acupuncture in alleviating menopausal discomforts, newborn abandonment, and intimate partner violence.

Lisa Jones Conley, RN, MS, NNP (author—Mormon chapter), is a neonatal nurse practitioner in the Newborn Intensive Care Unit at the University Hospitals and Clinics in Salt Lake City, UT. One of her interests has been in childbearing and childbearing practices in Mormonism. She has published her work in the journal *Neonatal Network.*

Judy Edwards, RN, MPH (author—Native American chapter), has worked as the liaison for Indian health for the Utah Department of Health. She was active in policy development to achieve the established health priority of improving Indian health in Utah. She facilitates improved working relationships between the health department, tribal health programs, local health departments, and private sector providers. She works closely with the Legislature regarding public health policy and its implications for American Indians in Utah. She is the contact person for individuals or providers trying to access coverage of services under Indian Health Services or other federally designed programs to meet the needs of Indian clients, and to identify culturally sensitive providers.

Alan Flattmann (cover artist) is a recipient of the American Artist Art Masters Award, a national recognition that honors America's most outstanding and gifted artists. He has also been awarded the Master Pastelist distinction by the Pastel Society of America, and has won major awards in many national painting exhibitions. His work can be found in numerous private and corporate publications and is represented by Bryant Galleries.

Judith Fullerton, CNM, PhD, FACNM (associate editor), has been an active practitioner of nurse-midwifery for more than 30 years and has also served as an educator of nurse-midwifery, nursing, medical, and other graduate-level (master's and doctoral) health professional students throughout her career. A Fellow of the American College of Nurse-Midwives (ACNM), she was recognized in 1997 by the National Perinatal Association (NPA) for individual contributions to maternal and child health, received the Alumni of the Year Award from Wayne State University in 1998, and in 2000 was the recipient of the Hattie Hemschemeyer Award, the highest honor bestowed by the ACNM, for her continuous, outstanding contributions to the profession of midwifery and the health of women and infants. She is a well-published author, the recipient of numerous project and research grants, a nationally and internationally respected consultant in the fields of evaluation and women's health, and an expert in testing and research. Dr Fullerton served as the previous vice president of programs for NPA.

M. Christina Glick, MD, FAAP (associate editor/coauthor— Professional Competence: Cultural/Religious Efficacy and the Principles of Family-Centered Care), is a neonatologist who has had a lifelong interest in serving minority and underserved populations of the rural south. She completed her undergraduate training at the University of Southern Mississippi, her medical training and pediatric residency at the University of Mississippi Medical Center in Jackson, and a postdoctoral fellowship in neonatology at the University of Texas Health Sciences Center in Houston. Currently she maintains a clinical appointment at the University of Mississippi Medical Center where she continues to supervise some research and occasionally takes call for the Neonatal Intensive Care Unit. She has also joined Newborn Associates, a group of neonatologists that serve several hospitals in the central part of Mississippi. Dr Glick assumed the presidency of the National Perinatal Association (NPA) on January 1, 2003, and is eager to expand NPA's visibility for maternal infant advocacy during her 2-year tenure. She will also continue in her role as director of transcultural development for NPA and will be working with a group of volunteers and employees on the completion of NPA's train the trainer program, *Transcultural Education: A Journey to Competence.*

Iffath Abbasi Hoskins, MD (author—Pakistani chapter), is currently the executive director of women's and children's services at Memorial Health University Medical Center. She is also a legal reviewer and consultant in risk management in the United States Navy. She is a tenured associate professor at New York University, Medical Center, Department of Obstetrics and Gynecology. She is on the board of directors of the Greater New York March of Dimes chapter. Dr Hoskins has recently been called to active duty for operation Noble Eagle.

Karen K. House, MSN, RNP (author—Seventh-Day Adventist chapter), has been a nurse practitioner (NP) in obstetrics and gynecology (OB/GYN) since the late 1970s. She attended Seventh-Day Adventist schools from first grade through graduate school. Currently she is working for Northern California Kaiser as an OB/GYN NP.

Lily S.Y. Hsia, CNM, MS, CPNP, FACNM (coauthor—Chinese chapter), is a certified nurse-midwife and certified pediatric nurse practitioner who has served on the faculty of the State University of

New York Downstate Medical Center since 1965 and chaired the Midwifery Education Program from 1988 until she retired in 2002. She currently works as a nursing and midwifery consultant for several education programs nationally and internationally and practices in an obstetrics and gynecology outreach clinic in New York City's Chinatown for St Vincent's Hospital. She was inducted as a Fellow of the American College of Nurse-Midwives in 1994 and has received many other awards and honors from her university and professional associations.

Shigeko Ito, PhD (coauthor—Japanese chapter), was born and reared in Japan. She attended Japanese schools from preschool through college, and then came to the United States in 1983 to pursue higher education. She received her doctorate in 1997 from the Stanford University School of Education. Her research interests focus on child development, early childhood education, issues relating to parenting and child-rearing practices, and cross-cultural differences between the United States and Japan regarding these topics.

Cheryl Killion, PhD, RN (author—African American chapter), a nurse and an anthropologist, is the director of the Center for Minority Family Health, School of Nursing at Hampton University in Hampton, Virginia. Her clinical and research background centers on women's health, with an emphasis on populations of African descent. She has conducted federally funded research on issues related to the intersection of gender, ethnicity, and social position. Her investigations have taken place in urban areas of the United States and in Belize. She has served as a consultant to the Pan American World Health Organization and collaborated with this organization to develop a videotape, "Innovations in Mental Health in Belize." Dr Killion has been a faculty member at the University of California at Los Angeles and the University of Michigan, where she developed and taught courses on cultural aspects of health and illness and complementary/alternative healing.

Yu-Ling Lai, RNC, MSN, CNS, CCRC (coauthor—Chinese chapter), was born in Taiwan and received her early professional training there. She is fluent in English, Chinese, and Taiwanese. She has had a broad range of clinical experience in both her native land and in the United States. She coordinates and conducts research for the University of Medicine and Dentistry of New Jersey/Robert Wood Johnson Medical School in the Division of Maternal-Fetal Medicine at St Peter's University Hospital.

Aleida Llanes-Oberstein, CNM, MS (author—Cuban chapter) is a graduate of Columbia University's Nurse-Midwifery Program, has been an assistant professor at the State University of New York Downstate Medical Center Midwifery Education Program since 1990, and has worked in a variety of clinical midwifery settings. Throughout her career, she has been an active member of the American College of Nurse-Midwives, both nationally and locally. She was appointed by the New York State Board of Regents to the New York State Board of Midwifery and currently serves as a board member. Through grant funding, Professor Llanes-Oberstein returned to her native Cuba leading a delegation of midwifery students and midwives, where they experienced the Cuban health care system firsthand by providing full-scope obstetric and gynecologic services to Cuban women. She was the first recipient of the Eugene B. Feigelson Presidential Outstanding Project Award for her work in Cuba.

Patricia Lozada-Santone, PhD (coauthor—Mexican chapter), holds a bachelor of science degree in health science and education and an MPH in maternal and child health. She received her doctorate degree from Claremont Graduate University. She is a founding member of the California Statewide Hispanic/Latino Tobacco Education Network based at University of Southern California. Dr Lozada-Santone is the vice president of the Latino caucus of the American Public Health Association. She serves on several national advisory committees related to public health issues for the Hispanic population. In addition, she has extensive experience in administration, education, and advocacy in this area.

Cheryl Major, RNC, BSN (Project "Birth Mother"), is the director of the Neonatal Outreach Program. Her duties include perinatal professional education and critical care transport. She is president-elect of the Tennessee Perinatal Association and is president of the Middle Tennessee Neonatal Nurses. Her dedication and determination to promote culturally competent care to all families gave impetus to the development of this transcultural resource guide.

Carole Ann Moleti, RNC, CNM, MS, MPH (author—Cambodian chapter), received a BS in nursing from Herbert H. Lehman College in the Bronx, NY, a master of science degree in nurse-midwifery, and an MPH in health administration from Columbia University. She has worked in women's health since 1979 in a variety of roles and settings and most recently as a family nurse practitioner and nurse-midwife. She has developed her interest and expertise in the care of socially high-risk women through her service in medically underserved areas such as Harlem, the South Bronx, and Washington Heights. Her work with medically underserved and minority women and their families has been published and presented at national conferences.

Renee B. Neri, RN, MS (author—Hmong chapter), is the director of community medical services at Women and Infants Hospital of Rhode Island. She coordinates and supervises community outreach activities, including the development and implementation of programs. Her community has a large number of non-English speaking women and therefore she has produced a series of culturally sensitive videotapes on 7 significant health topics that have been translated into 8 languages. She is also the clinical coordinator for a partnership program between Women and Infants Hospital and the University Hospital for obstetrics and gynecology in Tirana, Albania.

Sachiko Oshio, CNM, PhD (coauthor—Japanese chapter), currently is a clinical assistant professor at the University of Washington, School of Nursing and cares for Japanese women at the Nadeshiko Clinic. She was educated as a nurse-midwife in Japan and the United States and she taught in the nurse-midwifery graduate education program at the University of Washington, School of Nursing from 1994 to June 2000. She owns and operates a full-scope midwifery practice, lactation support, and educational services for Japanese-speaking clients in the Seattle/Puget Sound area. She is the author of a women's health handbook for Japanese women living in the United States. This book is written in Japanese and the content covers pregnancy, birth, lactation, and other useful information related to women's health.

Stuart Pickell, MD, MDiv (author—Spiritual Competence: Addressing Spirituality in the Medical Encounter) is a physician and a Presbyterian minister. Board certified in internal medicine and pediatrics, he practices in Fort Worth, TX, where he also serves as a parish associate at the First Presbyterian Church. He holds degrees in history from William and Mary College, theology from Princeton Theological Seminary, and medicine from the University of Texas—Southwestern Medical School in Dallas. Ordained in the Presbyterian Church (USA) in 1987, he served the church full time for 5 years before beginning his medical studies. He has served in leadership positions in the Presbyterian church as well as in the American Academy of Pediatrics and has published articles in both medical and religious journals. Dr Pickell carries his interest in spirituality into his medical practice, especially its effect on health and healing.

Mary Ann Shah, CNM, MS, FACNM (editor in chief), is president of the American College of Nurse-Midwives (ACNM). She is a Distinguished Fellow of ACNM and was honored by the organization in 1997 as the recipient of the Hattie Hemschemeyer Award, the highest honor it confers, and again in 2000 as Editor Emeritus following a 25-year career as editor in chief of the *Journal of Nurse-Midwifery*

(JNM)/Journal of Midwifery & Women's Health (JMWH). In 2003 JMWH established an annual writing award in her name. She also received an Alumni Achievement Award from Fordham University (1999), an award for individual contribution to maternal and child health from the National Perinatal Association (2000), and the Eugene B. Feigelson Award for dedicated leadership in advancing midwifery from The State University of New York Health Science Center at Brooklyn (2001). Ms Shah wrote the initial grant proposal that funded the Georgetown University nurse-midwifery education program, which flourishes to this day; pioneered a human sexuality education program for 5- to 21-year-old physically and cognitively challenged students; coordinated the first midwifery education program for non-nurses to be ACNM accredited and state approved; is a certified childbirth educator; and contributes to the perinatal health of families through the authorship and editing of health professional literature.

Ellen Shuzman, PhD, RN, BC, CNAA (author—Jewish chapter), is currently a clinical assistant professor at Rutgers, The State University of New Jersey, College of Nursing. She is responsible for theoretical and clinical curriculum and practice in childbearing, as well as leadership and management skills, in the baccalaureate program. She also serves as a nurse educator at the Northwest New Jersey Maternal and Child Health Network, responsible for planning and providing educational programs for professional nurses and other health care providers. In addition, Dr Shuzman has clinical expertise in the complementary healing modalities of therapeutic touch and relaxation techniques. She has had a longtime interest and has spoken often on the Jewish culture and its impact on health.

Luella Stiel, RNC, MSN (author—Cultural Competence: An Overview; Korean chapter), has 31 years of experience in perinatal nursing and 11 years of teaching in maternal/child nursing. Her practice is at the Macon Northside Hospital, the Baby Garden in Macon, GA.

Jane S. Wenger, RN, MSN, CRNP (author—Old Order Amish chapter), is a staff nurse in the cardiac critical care unit at the Good Samaritan Hospital and works in the emergency department at the Penn State Geisinger Health Care System, Milton S. Hershey Medical Center in Hershey, PA. Her research interest has been the Old Order Amish in Pennsylvania, and she has published her work on that population.

Disclaimer

This resource guide on the transcultural aspects of perinatal health care is designed to familiarize health care providers with a variety of cultural/religious traditions, beliefs, and practices that they might encounter in the care of women, infants, and families. No attempt has been made to pass any value judgments or censor the content presented. As such, the publication of any controversial material herein does not necessarily imply an endorsement by the National Perinatal Association or the American Academy of Pediatrics.

Volunteers who received no financial remuneration contributed the chapters that follow. Although great care has been taken to ensure the accuracy of all content and citations, some of the information presented may apply to specific subgroups of cultures, particular geographic locations, or certain generations; thus the currency and applicability of the material contained herein cannot be guaranteed. Additionally, individual or specific family cultural attributes may represent a blending or consolidation of several traditional and "Americanized" cultural practices.

Where appropriate, references are provided at the end of each section, both for attribution to the original sources and to enable those readers who are interested to read in greater depth about a given cultural/religious group. This publication is designed to foster awareness of the cultural complexities that may relate to the perinatal field and to serve as a handy reference for busy clinicians. As such, material is presented in a combination of narrative and outline form, providing detailed and quick answers to common questions regarding cultural and/or religious beliefs and traditions of selected populations.

Preface

Mary Ann Shah

According to the US Central Intelligence Agency's *World Factbook 2001*,[1] the United States ranked poorer in infant mortality than 39 other nations in the world with its reported 6.76 deaths per 1,000 live births. (See Table 1.) Even more startling are the 1999 comparative data[2] for white and African American populations (5.8 vs 14.6 infant deaths per 1,000 live births, respectively). These unacceptably high infant mortality rates are particularly troubling because they are attributable, in large part, to low birth weight (LBW), despite the fact that scientific evidence clearly shows that many of the antecedents and correlates of LBW are amenable to intervention through prenatal care. Of even greater concern are the March of Dimes' (MOD) estimates that prematurity in the United States increased more than 9% between 1990 and 2000 and that preterm babies accounted for 11.6% of the more than 4 million births in 2000.[3] The MOD[3] further reports that the rate of preterm birth in the United States is highest for African Americans (17.4%), followed by Native Americans (12.6%), Hispanics (11.4%), whites (10.6%), and Asians (10.2%).

In recognition of the disparities that exist in perinatal outcomes, Objective 16-1c of Healthy People 2010 recommends the reduction of infant deaths to 4.5 or fewer per 1,000 live births among all racial/ethnic groups.[4] Successful achievement of this goal will only be realized, however, by a 2-fold approach: increasing access to quality health care services for mothers and babies and a concomitant humanizing of the health care environment.

More promising data relate to women of Hispanic descent who comprised 11.2% of the US female population in 1999.[5] The infant

mortality rate attributed to this group for 1997 to 1999 was 5.8
per 1,000 live births.[2] In contrast, the 2001 infant mortality rates
for several Central and South American countries were dramatically
higher. For example, Guatemala, Peru, Brazil, Ecuador, and Nicaragua,
reported 45.79, 39.39, 36.96, 34.08, and 33.66 infant deaths per 1,000
live births, respectively.[1] (See Table 2.) Yet, it can probably be assumed
that the data for Latinas in the US include many who emigrated from
these very same nations and/or their offspring.

The United States is possibly the most culturally diversified nation
in the world. As such, US health care providers are all too often per-
plexed by the many cultural and/or religious beliefs and lifestyle practices that they encounter, particularly those that affect health indices.
Likewise, the impersonal bureaucracies associated with the Western
health care system can seem intimidating to those who immigrate to
the United States from distant shores. It must also be acknowledged
that the horrific events of September 11, 2001, have further sowed the
seeds of intercultural distrust, thereby negatively affecting the health
and security of the entire world.

Few can dispute the fact that a mutual lack of understanding
between providers of health care and immigrant patients exacerbates
communication barriers and leads to poor utilization of health services. Conversely, most would agree that "sensitivity and knowledge
of the patient's country of origin, health culture, and other related
norms, beliefs, and practices…can be effective at bridging the cultural gap that may prevent many immigrant women from seeking
preventative and curative care…."[6] While becoming culturally sensi-
tized, however, it is important to resist stereotyping people of any
particular national origin or religion, recognizing that within any
group, individuals, families, communities, and other subgroups can
differ substantially from one another in their beliefs and practices.
Moreover, adherence to cultural/religious traditions is often diminished through Western acculturation. Recommended standards for

culturally and linguistically appropriate health care services are presented in Table 3.[7]

While cultural and linguistic competencies have long been considered integral components of all health services,[8,9] this resource guide introduces 2 new concepts: those of professional and spiritual competencies, with the underlying premise that they are essential to any efforts to improve clinical outcomes for all women and families in the United States. For the purpose of clarity, the following definitions of terms will serve as the underpinnings of this resource guide on the transcultural aspects of perinatal health care:

- **Cultural Competence:** the awareness and respect for cultural/ religious practices, beliefs, and differences, enabling practitioners to adapt health care in accordance with the ethnocultural/religious heritage of the individual, family, and community[10]
- **Linguistic Competence:** the provision of bilingual staff or interpretation services for all clients without English language proficiency[7]
- **Professional Competence:** the accrual of scientific knowledge and skills and the application of the best evidence available in the rendering of health care that is congruent with the traditions and beliefs of members of diverse ethnocultural/religious groups
- **Spiritual Competence:** the ability to identify and understand one's own values and spiritual beliefs in the context of a pluralistic society, recognizing how interactions with patients and families may be affected by religious differences

The American Academy of Pediatrics (AAP) and the American College of Obstetricians and Gynecologists jointly recommend the provision of family-centered care that is sensitive to cultural diversity, preserves dignity, builds on strengths, offers real choices, and enhances competence.[11] Similarly, the American College of Nurse-Midwives advances the belief that "every family has a right to a safe, satisfying childbirth experience, with respect for cultural variations, human dignity and the rights as consumers to freedom of choice and self-determination."[12]

It must be emphasized that every belief system exists on a continuum, ranging from the most dogmatic to the least conventional practices; thus it behooves health care professionals to become knowledgeable about the cultural and spiritual commonalities that are prevalent within the communities they serve and to allow for any unique variations adopted by individual clients and families. Above all, the acquisition of cultural, professional, and spiritual competency must always be considered dynamic and evolutionary processes.

This resource guide was spearheaded by the National Perinatal Association and published by the AAP. Its purpose is to raise the consciousness of health care providers regarding the potential effect of culture and religion on the health and well-being of mothers, babies, and families. Because it would be virtually impossible to comprehensively feature each and every cultural and religious group that is represented in the United States, it is hoped that those presented herein will entice readers to independently research others through literature and online searches. For example, Gyamfi et al[13] have presented a praiseworthy model of obstetric care that is geared specifically to Jehovah's Witnesses, and it is anticipated that more and more exemplars of culturally competent care will become available in the near future. In the meantime, it is my honor to present to you the second edition of *Transcultural Aspects of Perinatal Health Care: A Resource Guide*. For further information, contact

National Perinatal Association
3500 E Fletcher Ave, Suite 205
Tampa, FL 33613
813/971-1008, 888/971-3295
Fax: 813/971-9306
E-mail: npa@nationalperinatal.org
www.nationalperinatal.org

Table 1
Infant Mortality of Nations With Rates Lower Than the United States*

Andorra:	4.08 deaths/1,000 live births (2001 est.)
Aruba:	6.39 deaths/1,000 live births (2001 est.)
Australia:	4.97 deaths/1,000 live births (2001 est.)
Austria:	4.44 deaths/1,000 live births (2001 est.)
Belgium:	4.7 deaths/1,000 live births (2001 est.)
Canada:	5.02 deaths/1,000 live births (2001 est.)
Czech Republic:	5.55 deaths/1,000 live births (2001 est.)
Denmark:	5.04 deaths/1,000 live births (2001 est.)
Finland:	3.79 deaths/1,000 live births (2001 est.)
France:	4.46 deaths/1,000 live births (2001 est.)
Germany:	4.71 deaths/1,000 live births (2001 est.)
Gibraltar:	5.49 deaths/1,000 live births (2001 est.)
Greece:	6.38 deaths/1,000 live births (2001 est.)
Guam:	6.71 deaths/1,000 live births (2001 est.)
Guernsey:	5 deaths/1,000 live births (2001 est.)
Hong Kong:	5.83 deaths/1,000 live births (2001 est.)
Iceland:	3.56 deaths/1,000 live births (2001 est.)
Ireland:	5.53 deaths/1,000 live births (2001 est.)
Italy:	5.84 deaths/1,000 live births (2001 est.)
Japan:	3.88 deaths/1,000 live births (2001 est.)
Jersey:	5.62 deaths/1,000 live births (2001 est.)
Liechtenstein:	4.99 deaths/1,000 live births (2001 est.)
Luxembourg:	4.77 deaths/1,000 live births (2001 est.)
Macau:	4.47 deaths/1,000 live births (2001 est.)
Malta:	5.83 deaths/1,000 live births (2001 est.)
Man, Isle of:	6.42 deaths/1,000 live births (2001 est.)
Monaco:	5.83 deaths/1,000 live births (2001 est.)
Netherlands:	4.37 deaths/1,000 live births (2001 est.)
New Zealand:	6.28 deaths/1,000 live births (2001 est.)
Northern Mariana Islands:	5.7 deaths/1,000 live births (2001 est.)
Norway:	3.94 deaths/1,000 live births (2001 est.)

Table 1
Infant Mortality of Nations With Rates Lower Than the United States*, continued

Portugal:	5.94 deaths/1,000 live births (2001 est.)
San Marino:	6.21 deaths/1,000 live births (2001 est.)
Singapore:	3.62 deaths/1,000 live births (2001 est.)
Slovenia:	4.51 deaths/1,000 live births (2001 est.)
Spain:	4.92 deaths/1,000 live births (2001 est.)
Sweden:	3.47 deaths/1,000 live births (2001 est.)
Switzerland:	4.48 deaths/1,000 live births (2001 est.)
United Kingdom:	5.54 deaths/1,000 live births (2001 est.)

*Source: US Central Intelligence Agency[1]

Table 2
Infant Mortality of Nations With Rates Higher Than the United States*

Afghanistan:	147.02 deaths/1,000 live births (2001 est.)
Albania:	39.99 deaths/1,000 live births (2001 est.)
Algeria:	40.56 deaths/1,000 live births (2001 est.)
American Samoa:	10.36 deaths/1,000 live births (2001 est.)
Angola:	193.72 deaths/1,000 live births (2001 est.)
Anguilla:	24.56 deaths/1,000 live births (2001 est.)
Antigua and Barbuda:	22.33 deaths/1,000 live births (2001 est.)
Argentina:	17.75 deaths/1,000 live births (2001 est.)
Armenia:	41.27 deaths/1,000 live births (2001 est.)
Azerbaijan:	83.08 deaths/1,000 live births (2001 est.)
Bahamas, The:	17.03 deaths/1,000 live births (2001 est.)
Bahrain:	19.77 deaths/1,000 live births (2001 est.)
Bangladesh:	69.85 deaths/1,000 live births (2001 est.)
Barbados:	12.04 deaths/1,000 live births (2001 est.)
Belarus:	14.38 deaths/1,000 live births (2001 est.)
Belize:	25.14 deaths/1,000 live births (2001 est.)
Benin:	89.68 deaths/1,000 live births (2001 est.)
Bermuda:	9.55 deaths/1,000 live births (2001 est.)
Bhutan:	108.89 deaths/1,000 live births (2001 est.)

Table 2
Infant Mortality of Nations With Rates Higher Than the United States*, *continued*

Bolivia:	58.98 deaths/1,000 live births (2001 est.)
Bosnia and Herzegovina:	24.35 deaths/1,000 live births (2001 est.)
Botswana:	63.2 deaths/1,000 live births (2001 est.)
Brazil:	36.96 deaths/1,000 live births (2001 est.)
British Virgin Islands:	20.3 deaths/1,000 live births (2001 est.)
Brunei:	14.4 deaths/1,000 live births (2001 est.)
Bulgaria:	14.65 deaths/1,000 live births (2001 est.)
Burkina Faso:	106.92 deaths/1,000 live births (2001 est.)
Burma:	73.71 deaths/1,000 live births (2001 est.)
Burundi:	70.74 deaths/1,000 live births (2001 est.)
Cambodia:	65.41 deaths/1,000 live births (2001 est.)
Cameroon:	69.83 deaths/1,000 live births (2001 est.)
Cape Verde:	53.22 deaths/1,000 live births (2001 est.)
Cayman Islands:	10.16 deaths/1,000 live births (2001 est.)
Central African Republic:	105.25 deaths/1,000 live births (2001 est.)
Chad:	95.06 deaths/1,000 live births (2001 est.)
Chile:	9.36 deaths/1,000 live births (2001 est.)
China:	28.08 deaths/1,000 live births (2001 est.)
Colombia:	23.96 deaths/1,000 live births (2001 est.)
Comoros:	84.07 deaths/1,000 live births (2001 est.)
Congo, Democratic Republic of the:	99.88 deaths/1,000 live births (2001 est.)
Congo, Republic of the:	99.73 deaths/1,000 live births (2001 est.)
Costa Rica:	11.18 deaths/1,000 live births (2001 est.)
Cote d'Ivoire:	93.65 deaths/1,000 live births (2001 est.)
Croatia:	7.21 deaths/1,000 live births (2001 est.)
Cuba:	7.39 deaths/1,000 live births (2001 est.)
Cyprus:	7.89 deaths/1,000 live births (2001 est.)
Djibouti:	101.51 deaths/1,000 live births (2001 est.)
Dominica:	16.54 deaths/1,000 live births (2001 est.)
Dominican Republic:	34.67 deaths/1,000 live births (2001 est.)

Table 2
Infant Mortality of Nations With Rates Higher Than the United States*, *continued*

Ecuador:	34.08 deaths/1,000 live births (2001 est.)
Egypt:	60.46 deaths/1,000 live births (2001 est.)
El Salvador:	28.4 deaths/1,000 live births (2001 est.)
Equatorial Guinea:	92.9 deaths/1,000 live births (2001 est.)
Eritrea:	75.14 deaths/1,000 live births (2001 est.)
Estonia:	12.62 deaths/1,000 live births (2001 est.)
Ethiopia:	99.96 deaths/1,000 live births (2001 est.)
Faroe Islands:	6.8 deaths/1,000 live births (2001 est.)
Fiji:	14.08 deaths/1,000 live births (2001 est.)
French Guiana:	13.61 deaths/1,000 live births (2001 est.)
French Polynesia:	9.12 deaths/1,000 live births (2001 est.)
Gabon:	94.91 deaths/1,000 live births (2001 est.)
Gambia, The:	77.84 deaths/1,000 live births (2001 est.)
Gaza Strip:	25.37 deaths/1,000 live births (2001 est.)
Georgia:	52.37 deaths/1,000 live births (2001 est.)
Ghana:	56.54 deaths/1,000 live births (2001 est.)
Greenland:	17.77 deaths/1,000 live births (2001 est.)
Grenada:	14.63 deaths/1,000 live births (2001 est.)
Guadalupe	9.53 deaths/1,000 live births (2001 est.)
Guatemala:	45.79 deaths/1,000 live births (2001 est.)
Guinea:	129.03 deaths/1,000 live births (2001 est.)
Guinea-Bissau:	110.4 deaths/1,000 live births (2001 est.)
Guyana:	38.72 deaths/1,000 live births (2001 est.)
Haiti:	95.23 deaths/1,000 live births (2001 est.)
Honduras:	30.88 deaths/1,000 live births (2001 est.)
Hungary:	8.96 deaths/1,000 live births (2001 est.)
India:	63.19 deaths/1,000 live births (2001 est.)
Indonesia:	40.91 deaths/1,000 live births (2001 est.)
Iran:	29.04 deaths/1,000 live births (2001 est.)
Iraq:	60.05 deaths/1,000 live births (2001 est.)
Israel:	7.72 deaths/1,000 live births (2001 est.)
Jamaica:	14.16 deaths/1,000 live births (2001 est.)

Table 2
Infant Mortality of Nations With Rates Higher Than the United States*, *continued*

Jordan:	20.36 deaths/1,000 live births (2001 est.)
Kazakhstan:	59.17 deaths/1,000 live births (2001 est.)
Kenya:	67.99 deaths/1,000 live births (2001 est.)
Kiribati:	54 deaths/1,000 live births (2001 est.)
Korea, North:	23.55 deaths/1,000 live births (2001 est.)
Korea, South:	7.71 deaths/1,000 live births (2001 est.)
Kuwait:	11.18 deaths/1,000 live births (2001 est.)
Kyrgyzstan:	76.5 deaths/1,000 live births (2001 est.)
Laos:	92.89 deaths/1,000 live births (2001 est.)
Latvia:	15.34 deaths/1,000 live births (2001 est.)
Lebanon:	28.35 deaths/1,000 live births (2001 est.)
Lesotho:	82.77 deaths/1,000 live births (2001 est.)
Liberia:	132.42 deaths/1,000 live births (2001 est.)
Libya:	28.99 deaths/1,000 live births (2001 est.)
Lithuania:	14.5 deaths/1,000 live births (2001 est.)
Macedonia	12.95 deaths/1,000 live births (2001 est.)
Madagascar:	83.58 deaths/1,000 live births (2001 est.)
Malawi:	121.12 deaths/1,000 live births (2001 est.)
Malaysia:	20.31 deaths/1,000 live births (2001 est.)
Maldives:	63.72 deaths/1,000 live births (2001 est.)
Mali:	121.44 deaths/1,000 live births (2001 est.)
Marshall Islands:	39.82 deaths/1,000 live births (2001 est.)
Martinique:	7.8 deaths/1,000 live births (2001 est.)
Mauritania:	76.7 deaths/1,000 live births (2001 est.)
Mauritius:	17.19 deaths/1,000 live births (2001 est.)
Mayotte:	69.54 deaths/1,000 live births (2001 est.)
Mexico:	25.36 deaths/1,000 live births (2001 est.)
Moldova:	42.74 deaths/1,000 live births (2001 est.)
Mongolia:	53.5 deaths/1,000 live births (2001 est.)
Montserrat:	8.19 deaths/1,000 live births (2001 est.)
Morocco:	48.11 deaths/1,000 live births (2001 est.)
Mozambique:	139.2 deaths/1,000 live births (2001 est.)

Table 2
Infant Mortality of Nations With Rates Higher Than the United States*, *continued*

Namibia:	71.66 deaths/1,000 live births (2001 est.)
Nauru:	10.71 deaths/1,000 live births (2001 est.)
Nepal:	74.14 deaths/1,000 live births (2001 est.)
Netherlands Antilles:	11.4 deaths/1,000 live births (2001 est.)
New Caledonia:	8.4 deaths/1,000 live births (2001 est.)
Nicaragua:	33.66 deaths/1,000 live births (2001 est.)
Niger:	123.57 deaths/1,000 live births (2001 est.)
Nigeria:	73.34 deaths/1,000 live births (2001 est.)
Oman:	22.52 deaths/1,000 live births (2001 est.)
Pakistan:	80.5 deaths/1,000 live births (2001 est.)
Palau:	16.67 deaths/1,000 live births (2001 est.)
Panama:	20.18 deaths/1,000 live births (2001 est.)
Papua New Guinea:	58.21 deaths/1,000 live births (2001 est.)
Paraguay:	29.78 deaths/1,000 live births (2001 est.)
Peru:	39.39 deaths/1,000 live births (2001 est.)
Philippines:	28.7 deaths/1,000 live births (2001 est.)
Poland:	9.39 deaths/1,000 live births (2001 est.)
Puerto Rico:	9.51 deaths/1,000 live births (2001 est.)
Qatar:	21.44 deaths/1,000 live births (2001 est.)
Reunion:	8.49 deaths/1,000 live births (2001 est.)
Romania:	19.36 deaths/1,000 live births (2001 est.)
Russia:	20.05 deaths/1,000 live births (2001 est.)
Rwanda:	118.92 deaths/1,000 live births (2001 est.)
Saint Helena:	22.38 deaths/1,000 live births (2001 est.)
Saint Kitts and Nevis:	16.28 deaths/1,000 live births (2001 est.)
Saint Lucia:	15.22 deaths/1,000 live births (2001 est.)
Saint Pierre and Miquelon:	8.39 deaths/1,000 live births (2001 est.)
Saint Vincent and the Grenadines:	16.61 deaths/1,000 live births (2001 est.)
Samoa:	31.75 deaths/1,000 live births (2001 est.)
Sao Tome and Principe:	48.96 deaths/1,000 live births (2001 est.)
Saudi Arabia:	51.25 deaths/1,000 live births (2001 est.)

Table 2
Infant Mortality of Nations With Rates Higher Than the United States*, *continued*

Senegal:	56.75 deaths/1,000 live births (2001 est.)
Seychelles:	17.3 deaths/1,000 live births (2001 est.)
Sierra Leone:	146.52 deaths/1,000 live births (2001 est.)
Slovakia:	8.97 deaths/1,000 live births (2001 est.)
Solomon Islands:	24.47 deaths/1,000 live births (2001 est.)
Somalia:	123.97 deaths/1,000 live births (2001 est.)
South Africa:	60.33 deaths/1,000 live births (2001 est.)
Sri Lanka:	16.08 deaths/1,000 live births (2001 est.)
Sudan:	68.67 deaths/1,000 live births (2001 est.)
Suriname:	24.27 deaths/1,000 live births (2001 est.)
Swaziland:	109.19 deaths/1,000 live births (2001 est.)
Syria:	33.8 deaths/1,000 live births (2001 est.)
Taiwan:	6.93 deaths/1,000 live births (2001 est.)
Tajikistan:	116.09 deaths/1,000 live births (2001 est.)
Tanzania:	79.41 deaths/1,000 live births (2001 est.)
Thailand:	30.49 deaths/1,000 live births (2001 est.)
Togo:	70.43 deaths/1,000 live births (2001 est.)
Tonga:	14.08 deaths/1,000 live births (2001 est.)
Trinidad and Tobago:	24.98 deaths/1,000 live births (2001 est.)
Tunisia:	29.04 deaths/1,000 live births (2001 est.)
Turkey:	47.34 deaths/1,000 live births (2001 est.)
Turkmenistan:	73.25 deaths/1,000 live births (2001 est.)
Turks and Caicos Islands:	18.06 deaths/1,000 live births (2001 est.)
Tuvalu:	22.65 deaths/1,000 live births (2001 est.)
Uganda:	91.3 deaths/1,000 live births (2001 est.)
Ukraine:	21.4 deaths/1,000 live births (2001 est.)
United Arab Emirates:	16.68 deaths/1,000 live births (2001 est.)
Uruguay:	14.7 deaths/1,000 live births (2001 est.)
Uzbekistan:	71.92 deaths/1,000 live births (2001 est.)
Vanuatu:	61.05 deaths/1,000 live births (2001 est.)
Venezuela:	25.37 deaths/1,000 live births (2001 est.)

Table 2
Infant Mortality of Nations With Rates Higher Than the United States*, *continued*

Vietnam:	30.24 deaths/1,000 live births (2001 est.)
Virgin Islands:	9.43 deaths/1,000 live births (2001 est.)
West Bank:	21.78 deaths/1,000 live births (2001 est.)
World:	52.61 deaths/1,000 live births (2001 est.)
Yemen:	68.53 deaths/1,000 live births (2001 est.)
Yugoslavia:	17.42 deaths/1,000 live births (2001 est.)
Zambia:	90.89 deaths/1,000 live births (2001 est.)
Zimbabwe:	62.61 deaths/1,000 live births (2001 est.)

*Source: US Central Intelligence Agency[1]

Table 3
Recommended Standards for Culturally and Linguistically Appropriate Health Care Services*

Preamble
Culture and language have considerable impact on how patients access and respond to health care services. To ensure equal access to quality health care by diverse populations, health care organizations and providers should

- Promote and support the attitudes, behaviors, knowledge, and skills necessary for staff to work respectfully and effectively with patients and each other in a culturally diverse work environment.
- Have a comprehensive management strategy to address culturally and linguistically appropriate services, including strategic goals, plans, policies, procedures, and designated staff responsible for implementation.
- Utilize formal mechanisms for community and consumer involvement in the design and execution of service delivery, including planning, policy making, operations, evaluation, training, and, as appropriate, treatment planning.
- Develop and implement a strategy to recruit, retain, and promote qualified, diverse, and culturally competent administrative, clinical, and support staff that are trained and qualified to address the needs of the racial and ethnic communities being served.
- Require and arrange for ongoing education and training for administrative, clinical, and support staff in culturally and linguistically competent service delivery.
- Provide all clients with limited English proficiency (LEP) access to bilingual staff or interpretation services.

**Table 3
Recommended Standards for Culturally and Linguistically Appropriate
Health Care Services*, *continued***

- Provide oral and written notices, including translated signage at key points of contact, to clients in their primary language informing them of their right to receive no cost interpreter services.
- Translate and make available signage and commonly used written patient educational material and other materials for members of the predominant language groups in service areas.
- Ensure that interpreters and bilingual staff can demonstrate bilingual proficiency and receive training that includes the skills and ethics of interpreting, and knowledge in both languages, of the terms and concepts relevant to clinical or nonclinical encounters. Family or friends are not considered adequate substitutes because they usually lack these abilities.
- Ensure that the clients' primary spoken language and self-identified race/ethnicity are included in the health care organization's management information system as well as any patient records used by provider staff.
- Use a variety of methods to collect and utilize accurate demographic, cultural, epidemiological, and clinical outcome data for racial and ethnic groups in the service area, and become informed about the ethnic/cultural needs, resources, and assets of the surrounding community.
- Undertake ongoing organizational self-assessments of cultural and linguistic competence, and integrate measures of access, satisfaction, quality, and outcomes for culturally and linguistically appropriate services (CLAS) into other organizational internal audits and performance improvement programs.
- Develop structures and procedures to address cross-cultural ethical and legal conflicts in health care delivery and complaints or grievances by patients and staff about unfair, culturally insensitive, or discriminatory treatment, or difficulty in accessing services, or denial of services.
- Prepare an annual progress report documenting the organizations' progress with implementing CLAS standards, including information on programs, staffing, and resources.

Source: US Department of Health and Human Services Office of Minority Health[7]

References

1. US Central Intelligence Agency. *World Factbook 2001*. Available at: http://www.bartleby.com/151/a28.html. Accessed February 15, 2003
2. Centers for Disease Control and Prevention. National Center for Health Statistics mortality data based on race of infant as numerator and race of mother as denominator. *MMWR Morb Mortal Wkly Rep.* 2002;51:589–592. Available at: http://www.cdc.gov/mmwr/preview/mmwrhtml1/mm5127a1.htm. Accessed February 15, 2003
3. March of Dimes. *2002 US Prematurity Profile*. Available at: http://www.marchofdimes.com/peristats. Accessed February 15, 2003
4. US Department of Health and Human Services. *Healthy People 2010* (Conference Edition, in 2 Volumes). Washington, DC: US Department of Health and Human Services; 2000
5. US Department of Health and Human Services, Office on Women's Health. *The Health of Minority Women*. Washington, DC: US Department of Health and Human Services; 2000. Available at: http://www.4woman.gov/owh/pub/minority/index.htm. Accessed February 15, 2003
6. The Maternal and Child Health Community Leadership Institute. *Understanding the Health Culture of Recent Immigrants to the United States: A Cross-Cultural Maternal Health Information Catalog*. Washington, DC: American Public Health Association. Available at: http://www.apha.org/ppp/red/Background.htm. Accessed February 15, 2003
7. US Department of Health and Human Services Office of Minority Health. *Assuring Cultural Competence in Health Care: Recommendations for National Statistics and an Outcomes-Focused Research Agenda*. Washington, DC: Available at: http://www.omhrc.gov/clas/ds.htm. Accessed February 15, 2003
8. Spector RE. *Cultural Diversity in Health & Illness*. 5th ed. Upper Saddle River, NJ: Prentice Hall Health; 2000
9. Rorie JL, Paine LL, Barger MK. Primary care for women: cultural competence in primary care services. *J Nurse Midwifery*. 1996;41:92–100
10. Spector RE. *CulturalCare: Guides to Heritage Assessment and Health Traditions*. 2nd ed. Upper Saddle River, NJ: Prentice Hall Health; 2000
11. American Academy of Pediatrics, American College of Obstetricians and Gynecologists. *Guidelines for Perinatal Care*. 5th ed. Elk Grove Village, IL: American Academy of Pediatrics and Washington, DC: American College of Obstetricians and Gynecologists; 2002

12. American College of Nurse-Midwives. *ACNM Statement on Practice Settings.* Washington, DC: American College of Nurse-Midwives; 1997
13. Gyamfi C, Mavis M, Gyamfi MM, Berkowitz RL. Ethical and medicolegal considerations in the obstetric care of a Jehovah's Witnesses. *Obstet Gynecol.* 2003;102:173–180

Foreword

Cheryl Major

Cultural diversity continues to be an evolving national issue and priority. The National Perinatal Association (NPA) embraces this priority in the fullest measure because of the implications for quality of life and health status for all populations.

Mission
NPA promotes the health and well-being of mothers and infants, thereby enriching families, communities, and our world.

Vision
NPA will engage the broadest possible coalition to improve social, cultural, and economic environments for optimal health and well-being of mothers, infants, and families.

Membership
Membership in NPA is open to any individual, organization, or corporation interested in perinatal health care. Members are representative of a variety of disciplines. Individuals and groups interested in improved physical, mental, and emotional stability of infants and their families come together to

- Ensure NPA can carry out effective relationship building, education, research, leadership, and advocacy.
- Work toward a common goal—better health care for mothers and infants.
- Focus on the issues rather than individual professions while being sensitive to medical and nonmedical values.
- Provide an opportunity for consumers and health professionals to work together.

- Help construct a national framework for advocacy of better health for infants and mothers.
- Help increase multidisciplinary involvement and understanding in perinatal health.
- Demonstrate a commitment to quality patient care and patients' rights.

Cultural diversity is a major emerging initiative across the United States. NPA continues to draw attention to this vital subject by means of conference speakers; articles in our newsletter, bulletin, and state association periodicals; and coalition building.

Relevance and Meaning: Transcultural Aspects of Perinatal Health Care

The portal through which improvement in the health status of financially impoverished communities can be initiated is that which starts with perinatal and maternal and child care. Reproduction and the activities surrounding childbirth have historically been greatly influenced by societal, religious, and cultural traditions. During the last 2 decades, there has been a movement throughout American society to promote greater cultural diversity, sensitivity, and competence, and this goal will become even more relevant in the next 20 years. A case in point, it is estimated that 1 in every 13 residents in the United States is foreign-born.[1] By 2010 it is projected that 1 in 10 residents will have hailed from a foreign country. United States census figures estimate that the number of US residents for whom English is a foreign language rose from 23 million in 1980 to 31.8 million in 1990.[2]

Providers of maternal and child health services have been at the forefront of advocating for culturally competent service delivery. Health is not just the absence of disease or infirmities; rather, it is the presence of social, emotional, economic, spiritual, environmental, and psychological well-being. Culture provides rules that govern a person's behavior, including how to promote, maintain, and restore one's health and coping strategies when faced with stress and crisis. Showing respect for the uniqueness of individuals and their culture is a requirement in a multicultural health care setting. Human beings have the right to be assessed and treated within the framework of their own cultural ways. Furthermore, ignorance of culture-specific information can alienate clients and decrease adherence to treatment plans. Caregivers must seek to maintain as many of the valued customs as possible or make adaptations as necessary, trying only to alter potentially harmful practices.

Culturally appropriate care increases the ability to ensure that the quality of life is maximized for present generations of mothers and children and ensures that the heritage of past, present, and future generations is preserved. The assumption that health care providers have general background information about particular cultural or religious groups living in their community is often erroneous. There is an urgent need for materials and programs to reduce the cultural gap between health care providers and their clients. To encourage mutual sensitivity, trust, and respect, clinicians need to understand different beliefs about pregnancy and maternity care. Toward that end, multidisciplinary and multicultural contributors developed this resource guide. The target audience includes anyone who interacts with families during pregnancy, childbirth, or the postpartum period. Thus clinics, public health departments, physician/midwife offices, birthing centers, hospitals, and academic programs would be key beneficiaries of this culture-specific information.

References

1. Purnell LD, Paulanka BJ. Transcultural diversity and health care. In: Purnell LD, Paulanka BJ, eds. *Transcultural Health Care: A Culturally Competent Approach*. Philadelphia, PA: FA Davis; 1998:1–51
2. Building bridges with words: medical interpreters cross the language barrier. *Opening Doors*. Fall 1995

Cultural Competence: An Overview

Luella Stiel

"Give me your tired, your poor,
Your huddled masses, yearning to breathe free,
The wretched refuse of your teeming shore.
Send these, the homeless, tempest-tost to me,
I lift my lamp beside the golden door!"
                              Emma Lazarus—*The New Colossus,* 1883

This famous inscription, found at the base of the Statue of Liberty,
reminds us of the significance of the United States as a refuge for
the oppressed from other lands. Immigrants come to this nation
with hopes and dreams, but most of all seeking freedom to be who
they are.

In the past decade 12 million new immigrants have come to the
United States, exceeding the largest previous wave of approximately
10 million immigrants between 1905 and 1914.[1] Often described as
a melting pot in which various cultures become blended, in reality,
immigrants to this country bring their individual cultures with them,
contributing to the society they have joined yet maintaining their
uniqueness. Being culturally sensitive is having the ability to recognize
and appreciate that diversity only enriches our cultural environment.

Among health professionals, there is increasing awareness that if
health care goals are to be met, care must be culturally appropriate.
Culturally inappropriate health care has been shown to be associated
with negative outcomes.[1] This is especially true of perinatal care. A
recurring theme of almost all cultures is the creation of rites and rituals around important life events.[2] No life events may be more important than pregnancy and childbirth. It makes sense, therefore, that

assisting health professionals to develop cultural competence and sensitivity should contribute greatly to the improvement of perinatal outcomes in the United States.

To be culturally competent is not to know everything there is to know about all cultures. Cultural competence is an educative process that involves developing self-awareness, learning to appreciate the difference and the value of cultural practices other than one's own, and having behavioral flexibility.[1] To become more culturally competent,[2] perinatal health care providers should strive to[2]:

1. Include cultural assessment as a routine part of perinatal health care.
2. Assess their own cultural beliefs, identifying personal biases, stereotypes, and prejudices.
3. Make a conscious commitment to respect and value the beliefs of others.
4. Learn the customs and rituals of the common cultural groups within the community.
5. Seek input from the client regarding her health-related traditions and practices.
6. Evaluate if what is about to be taught is really better than what the client is already doing for herself.
7. Adapt care to meet the special needs of the client and her family, as long as standards of health and safety are not compromised.

References

1. Lester N. Cultural competence: a nursing dialogue. *Am J Nurs.* 1998;98:26–33
2. Olds SB, London ML, Ladewig PW. *Maternal-Newborn Nursing: A Family Approach to Care.* 5th ed. New York, NY: Addison-Wesley; 1996

Professional Competence: Cultural/Religious Efficacy and the Principles of Family-Centered Care

Joseph J. Botti and M. Christina Glick

"Diverse—Anyone who is not you."

Ana Núñez, MD

The chronicle of this nation's evolving identity is an account of conflict and compassion, of bigotry and tolerance, of interpopulation disorientation and gradual understanding. It is quite likely that no other country has ever experienced as much change in its psychosocial, economic, and cultural/religious makeup over so short a historic period as has the United States. Our national legacy is the recognition of men, women, and children of all colors, creeds, national origins, and socioeconomic status as equal. In health care, the emergence of culturally, spiritually, and professionally sensitive attitudes toward the clinical needs of individuals and families from diverse cultures reflects our national cultural evolution, warts and all. Within academic circles, there is a growing consensus that health professionals should possess the attitudes, behaviors, and skills that will eliminate cultural barriers to promoting health, preventing disease, and providing optimal care for all patients and their families.

It must be emphasized that there are, as yet, no specific yardsticks for demonstrating "professional competence" within the health care arena and that acquiring aptitude sufficient to satisfy a universal benchmark requires an agreed-to evaluation process. Many professions are undergoing self-examination, anticipating that common barometers will eventually be realized. In the meantime, a solid foundation for the care of families with diverse cultural backgrounds should encompass 5 elements: specialized knowledge, competent skills, high ethical standards, accountability, cultural/spiritual competence, and a predilection toward family-centered care.

Because the practice of professional competency is fundamentally intertwined with adopting culturally and spiritually competent behaviors, the teaching of all 3 should be considered to complement one another. However, 2 recent studies have found that many traditionally cherished values, such as honesty, altruism, non-malfeasance, and confidentiality, are no longer an integral part of curricula that "teach" professionalism.[1,2] The following questions are, thus, offered as the basis for developing professional competency:

1. What are the anticipated behaviors of specific cultural/religious groups that are likely to be undertaken in the context of health promotion and disease prevention?
2. How critical are these particular traditions in the health decisions to be made?
3. What are the general standards of safety, security, and public health that may affect culturally/spiritually sensitive interactions with families?
4. How can faith ministers assist in resolving spiritual issues that may affect family decision making?
5. What alternative interactions may be considered that might be accepted as non-harmful or helpful in the context of specific clinical situations?
6. What characteristics do health professionals need to demonstrate when caring for culturally and religiously diverse patients and their families?
7. How can communities and their members become a part of the structure of health care, serving as partners in the ongoing learning curve required for culturally/spiritually competent medical decision making?

Culturally/religiously appropriate health care encounters start with a willingness of the provider to engage in a mutually respectful relationship with patients and their families. It is expected that the provider begins with a sound scientific basis for practice and a strong foundation in medical/ethical thinking. Decisions by health professionals should be, by nature, other-focused, based on benevolence and respectful of the patient. The benevolent characteristics of ethical decision making by health professionals include the following virtues: self-effacement, self-sacrifice, compassion, and integrity.[3] As these virtues are translated into practical professional attributes, it is important to recognize that the values, goals, and priorities that individuals and families from diverse cultural backgrounds bring to the clinical interaction have a profound effect on the relationship.

Integral to developing professionalism, transcultural competency, and family-centered care is the incorporation of family and community representation within the health care team. Although this can be a threatening concept to providers, it is a necessary component for ensuring quality health care services, favorable outcomes of disease, overall good health, and positive health care experiences. Inviting patients or their advocates/surrogates to become partners in the health care team can provide direction to caregivers, facilitate shared decision making, promote mutual understanding and cooperation, and enhance the development of competency standards.

Defining cultural competence requires a workable definition of culture. In light of the more than 150 definitions of culture,[4] Núñez[5] explains the nature of culture in terms of what it does rather than what it is. "Culture shapes how we explain and value our world. Culture is the lens through which we give our world meaning. Culture shapes our beliefs and influences our behaviors about what is appropriate…. The skill of using multiple cultural lenses is called 'cultural competence.'"[5] From a more institutional view, cultural competence may be viewed as "a set of academic and interpersonal skills that allow individuals to increase their understanding and appreciation of cultural differences and similarities, within, among, and between groups."[6]

Núñez[5] further suggests that for the caregiver to be effective in interactions involving individuals and families of different cultures, the idea of cross-cultural efficacy should be promoted, implying that neither the caregiver's nor the patient's culture should hold sway, but that a balanced tricultural collaboration, including the respective personal cultural values of the provider, the patient (family), and the culture of medical professionalism, needs to be negotiated, affirmed, and translated into mutually agreeable health decisions. Thereby the interaction becomes ethno-relative rather than ethnocentric. Several professional attributes should be employed within the context of the tricultural health/medical interaction.

The first attribute is an awareness of the patient's cultural values, recognizing that it is virtually impossible for any health professional to have a clear a priori awareness of the cultural dynamics of each family with whom he or she interacts. The underlying principle of awareness, then, is to acknowledge our own limited understanding of how families address health issues in the context of their cultural foundations. To gain such awareness requires that we seek information from patients about their cultural environments and what they perceive to be important, but negotiable, versus nonnegotiable values of their medical and health behaviors and decision making. To determine the unique cultural environment of each family, we might ask a leading question such as: "What would you like me to know about your family traditions and beliefs (culture, faith) so that I can best help you when making medical decisions?"

The second attribute is self-awareness. Each of us brings culturally derived assumptions, prejudices, and experiences to each clinical interaction; thus awareness of our own cultural values is a necessary step in the journey to cultural/spiritual and professional competence. In our continually changing society, prejudgments about cultural and religious principles or beliefs are inappropriate. Self-awareness is the intellectual corollary to the medical/ethical virtue of self-effacement; it provides a touchstone for initiating fair deliberative interactions with our patients and helps us to identify values and beliefs that affect priorities, goals, and visions for the family.

Cultural humility is the third attribute. This involves a lifelong commitment to self-evaluation and self-critique, to redressing the power imbalances in the patient/physician dynamic, and to developing mutually beneficial and non-paternalistic clinical and advocacy partnerships with individuals/families/communities from diverse populations.[7] Attainment of cultural humility rejects ethnocentric views and shuns the one-dimensional thinking that often exists within our health culture.

Cultural/religious efficacy represents the final attribute that can foster professional competency. Through an interactive process of reciprocity,[8] the inequities of power can be ameliorated between health care providers (physicians, midwives, nurses, social service/ public health personnel), and consumers (patients and their families). To be successful in this endeavor, however, health care providers must be able to

1. Acknowledge any differences between their own cultural/spiritual values and those of the patient/family with whom they are interacting.
2. Foster mutual respect and understanding.
3. Determine the most effective way of adapting professional interpretations and recommendations to the value system of each family.
4. Provide safe and realistic choices to patients/families within the least restrictive environment.
5. Promote equity for all, no matter what the cultural/religious background.

Cultures must be viewed as dynamic with changes occurring over time and as a result of emigration. Each member of every culture brings their own individual and unique interpretation of the culture and, therefore, understanding the practice of one member does not guarantee understanding and knowledge of the next patient from the same culture. The following "cultural" vital signs should be explored during each encounter in the health care setting:

- The role of extended family members and their traditions in decisions
- The role of community or religious leaders in decision making and health practices
- The role of gender within the family
- Practices and traditions around health and health care and specific perinatal practices
- Dietary issues

Similarly, health professionals need to stay true to their own beliefs within the context of scientific data and, above all, abide by the "do no harm" principle and follow the dictates of evidence-based practice. Unfortunately, conflicts may arise between sound medical standards and cultural/religious practices or beliefs, negatively affecting the interactions between health professionals and families. These are extremely difficult situations with which to deal, particularly when the conflict may not be resolvable. Nevertheless, it is imperative for providers to strive to negotiate the best resolution while attempting to maintain a functional interaction with the patient and family. Although preserving the health and welfare of the patient and family is always paramount, disrespect should never be shown.

Cultural/spiritual and professional competencies are becoming increasingly interdependent in our diverse and complicated health care system. In addition to the changing environments of the world in which we live and work, there are increasing demands from all segments of the population to more sensitively accommodate alternative traditions, lifestyles, and beliefs. Health care providers are faced with the added dilemma of balancing the teachings and ethics of their respective professions with the sometimes conflicting expectations of their patients. They must learn to negotiate a compromise that balances both sets of values so that successful health partnerships can be achieved between themselves and the individuals and families for whom they care.

References

1. Cruess SR, Cruess RL. Professionalism must be taught. *Brit Med J.* 1997;315:1674–1677
2. Stern DT. Values on call: a method for assessing the teaching of professionalism. *Acad Med.* 1996;17(Suppl):537–539
3. McCullough LB, Chervanek FA. *Ethics in Obstetrics and Gynecology.* New York, NY: Oxford University Press; 1994
4. Kroeber AL, Kluckhorn C. *Culture: A Critical Review of Concepts and Definitions.* New York, NY: Vintage Books; 1952
5. Núñez AE. Transforming cultural competence into cross-cultural efficacy in women's health education. *Acad Med.* 2000;75:1071–1080
6. US Department of Health and Human Services. *Cultural Competence for Evaluators: A Guide for Alcohol and Other Drug Abuse Prevention Practitioners Working With Ethnic/Racial Communities.* Rockville, MD: US Department of Health and Human Services; 1992
7. Tervalon M, Murray-Garcia J. Cultural humility versus cultural competence: a critical distinction in defining physician training outcomes in multicultural education. *J Health Care Poor Underserved.* 1998;9:117–125
8. Harry B, Day M, Kalyanpur M. Cultural reciprocity in sociocultural perspective: adapting the normalization principle for family collaboration. *Exceptional Child.* 1999;66:123–136

Spiritual Competence: Addressing Spirituality in the Medical Encounter

Stuart Pickell

Most religions of the world address the fundamental questions about what it means to be human. While varying in their orientation, many explore the unique interrelationships that exist between body, mind, and spirit, recognizing that a condition that affects one part affects every part. This is one of the great contributions that religion makes to health care. However, health care providers face a difficult challenge. On the one hand, they must acknowledge the importance of religion to themselves and to their patients; on the other hand, their medical training tends to emphasize objectivity and encourages them to leave religion out of their encounters with patients and their families.

This has not always been the case. Historically, religion and medicine were inseparably linked. The religious leaders of various sects and tribal religions functioned as healers of body, mind, and spirit. In some circles, they still do. However, during the last 500 years, medicine and religion have parted ways. The emphasis on scientific reasoning during the past 2 centuries and the emergence of a general distrust of anything that cannot be empirically proven have reinforced this artificial division. What evolved was an environment in which health care professionals who wanted to care for their patients holistically were impeded by the view that the spiritual dimension was beyond their domain and that to address religious beliefs would be professionally inappropriate. Recently, however, we have come to realize that failure to address spiritual concerns means ignoring issues that are profoundly important and relevant to health care.

Since September 11, 2001, the important role that religion plays in the lives of individuals as well as in geopolitical affairs has become very evident; however, the relationship between religious beliefs and health care practices may not be quite so clear. In the Judeo-Christian tradition, for example, the word "shalom," loosely translated "peace," more accurately refers to an inner peace characterized by wholeness in body, mind, and spirit. This presupposes that an individual is a person, and not just a body, to be healed, even if cure is impossible. This is true, of course, for many other religions as well. In other words, the traditions of religion and healing must be viewed as inextricably intertwined.

This resource guide is designed to help health care providers understand the role religion plays in health care in a variety of cultural and religious contexts. It's not enough simply to know that religion is important; we must know *how* it is important. This deeper level of understanding requires that we know not just the corporate traditional values held by our patients' socioreligious groups, but also how our patients express these values in their own lives. Only by learning about the religious traditions from which our patients come, and then understanding how our patients assimilate these traditions, can we truly assist our patients on the road to healing. The goal is that by acquiring this understanding we will become more "spiritually competent."

Spiritual competency goes hand in hand with cultural and professional competency. In the former, we recognize the importance of understanding the cultural milieu in which people live and the traditions that define their lives. In the latter, we acknowledge the importance of having adequate and appropriate technologic training and equipment. But in the end we realize that treating the whole person competently requires more than just an understanding of their culture or a mastery of our profession. It requires that we incorporate the values that our patients deem significant in the healing process. Being spiritually competent, however, does not end with an understanding of our patients and their religious beliefs. It also requires a modicum of self-understanding. It requires that we know our own beliefs and biases and how they affect our relationships with our patients. We must always be open to the question: How might our beliefs interfere with our patient's journey toward healing?

Learning how to address spiritual issues with our patients can be a daunting task, even for those who are comfortable talking about spirituality. Historic precedent would dictate that health care practitioners only address issues related to the physical body and the life sciences that govern it, the assumption being that spiritual issues are better left to religious professionals.

Some have gone so far as to argue that engaging our patients in conversations regarding their spiritual preferences or practices may even hurt our patients as they may read into them some hint of guilt or moral flaw that resulted in their current predicament. Such a view, however, fails to give credit to the patient as an independent and autonomous, much less spiritual, being capable of rejecting such a conversation. It also fails to give credit to the health care provider who is seeking to help the patient by bringing into the healing process resources beyond the realm of traditional medicine. We must always remember that our ultimate responsibility is to the patient. And healing, in our patient's mind, may include some religious elements. We must listen to them and try to understand how religion influences their beliefs and, if possible, incorporate these practices into the healing process. After all, we are not treating diseases; we are treating people *with* diseases.

Anyone who has spent a significant amount of time in a hospital has seen the relative ease that many clergy and religious professionals have in a hospital environment. This stems, at least in part, from the traditional role that the clergy has always had as healers of the whole person. Many religious professionals recognize that at the core of their ministry is the hope that the beliefs they espouse will ultimately help their charges find inner peace—shalom—wholeness. It's what they do every day, everywhere. The hospital is merely another location wherein healing takes place. The hospital's importance is heightened, however, by the fact that the physical needs are much more acute there, thus bringing the spiritual needs closer to the surface. What clergy seek for their charges then is different from what health care providers tend to seek. Health care providers tend to seek only a cure whereas clergy seek healing, whether a cure is a realistic possibility.

Although many clergy are comfortable in the medical environment, most are not equipped to interpret or even address the medical issues and nuances presented by the patient. This task lies squarely with the "professionally competent" medical professional. However, as health care providers, we must not restrict our focus to medical topics. We must be willing to reach across the line that has divided medicine and religion and try to incorporate the religious beliefs and/or practices of our patients into the overall plan for their care. It is certainly acceptable, therefore, to broach the area of religious beliefs in the context of a medical encounter, and many of our patients will appreciate the gesture. At the very least, we must make an effort to understand these beliefs to anticipate potential conflicts that may come between our patients and their recovery or treatment. We must create an environment that is "spiritually" friendly. Indeed, we must practice hospitality in our hospitals and other health care settings as we strive to welcome the religious practices of our patients so that they can incorporate their own traditions into the healing process.

There may be instances, however, when a patient's religious practices or medical requests pose an ethical dilemma, as characterized by the following 3 general scenarios:

- A patient wants to engage in a religious practice that the health care provider believes interferes with the accepted standard of care.
- A patient makes a medical request that the health care provider considers objectionable on moral or religious grounds.

- A patient wants to engage in a religious practice that the health care provider considers objectionable on moral or religious grounds.

All 3 scenarios involve religious beliefs or practices, but in 2 of the scenarios the provider's religious beliefs are part of the equation. Thus it is clear that addressing these issues requires maturity, self-awareness, and objectivity.

In the first scenario, the religious practice is contrary to the accepted standard of care. Before responding, the health care provider must assess the risk posed by the patient's practice and seek to understand the patient's spiritual orientation. Understanding what the practice is gets us half way there, but it also helps to understand the significance it holds for the patient with reference to spiritual and physical healing. Once understood, we must identify what it is about their belief that is incongruous with appropriate medical care and discern whether a danger truly exists or if it merely represents our bias or distaste for the practice.

A prima facie rule of medical ethics is that health care providers must promote patient autonomy in making health care decisions. The role of the provider is to inform, not influence. If we are to promote and respect patient autonomy, we must honor the patient's decisions. A classic example is that of a Jehovah's Witness patient who refuses a potentially life-saving blood transfusion. Assuming that the patient is an adult, the provider is obligated to honor the patient's request that no blood products be given. Rare exceptions, usually involving minors,* can cloud the issue, but for the most part, this is an honorable goal.

---

*The scenario wherein the patient is a minor and the parents are Jehovah's Witnesses raises an entirely different set of questions. Here, the religious beliefs and rights of the parent are weighed against the inherent right to life of the patient, a minor child, who presumably is not old enough to act on his or her own behalf. Furthermore, the state has an obligation to protect the child from capricious acts or decisions made by the parents that might threaten the life of the child. Questions involving minors become more tenuous because legal statutes and precedents are involved.

In the second scenario, the patient seeks a medical procedure that is legal and for which medical standards of care exist. We presume that the provider is trained to provide the procedure but refuses on moral or religious grounds. An example might be a 19-year-old woman in her first trimester of pregnancy who requests an abortion from a gynecologist who opposes abortion. The provider is not obligated to provide elective procedures; she or he is certainly within her or his right not to perform the procedure. Whether the provider refers the patient to someone who will, on the other hand, is another issue.

In the third scenario, a patient wishes to engage in an unconventional practice that the provider finds objectionable for religious, not medical, reasons. An example might involve a Wiccan patient who wishes to engage in a healing ritual in her hospital room. What if her provider, a conservative Christian, considers the Wiccan religion to be tantamount to witchcraft and regards the ritual both difficult to understand and objectionable on religious grounds? In this case, she or he may want to take a step back and reassess the situation in light of what we now know about spirituality competency. In other words, rather than imposing our beliefs or value systems on patients, we must help them to utilize their own beliefs and value systems in an effort to facilitate healing, even if we do not comprehend or agree with these beliefs or practices. In this scenario, because there is no medical contraindication, it would be reasonable for the provider to try to accommodate the practice within the confines of the safety regulations of the institution.

While we cannot, in good conscience, behave in a manner that is contrary to our own value systems, we can do whatever is in our power to assist the patient in locating the necessary resources—even another provider who is willing to offer traditional medical care in the midst of non-traditional healing endeavors. The key here is to avoid becoming a hindrance to a patient's healing, including spiritual healing. Again, this requires that we know our own beliefs and understand how we are influenced by our own biases and prejudices. We also need to recognize the interplay and possible tensions that may exist between our views and those held by the patient. While the potential for ethical dilemmas still exists, this approach differs from that posited by medical ethicists because it explores the importance of religion to individuals and not just to their cultural groups.

Medical ethicists tend to work outside the religious arena in an effort to be unbiased and to present ethical principles that have global or universal relevance. Thus they focus on common or universally held values and understandings that are morally justifiable and medically responsible. Any reference to religion, therefore, is within the context of the greater corporate cultural traditions or beliefs. The problem with this approach—at least as it relates to this discussion— is that by operating outside of the religious arena, they circumvent the core value systems that most individuals draw on to form their opinions about what is morally justifiable. After all, the only principles that are relevant to patients are the ones that have meaning to them, the ones that have been shaped and molded, not just by the general beliefs and practices of their respective cultural group, but by their own unique interpretations and assimilations of those beliefs. If we don't make some effort to get at what these are, we miss out on a valuable opportunity to help a particular patient. And if we aren't aware of our own values and beliefs, we may inadvertently interfere with our patients' healing.

Once we understand that religion is important, we must find a way to ascertain if it is important to our patients and, if so, how. There are several ways a health care provider might introduce the subject of religion and spirituality with their patients, only one of which I will address here. Although the method I recommend is designed for a verbal conversation, it can be modified and used as an optional part of a patient questionnaire. Either way, the method is simple, easy to memorize, and will result in a nonthreatening interview in which all of the information needed regarding a patient's spiritual orientation can be obtained. It uses the mnemonic "FACT," which stands for the following:

- **Faith:** Does religious faith or spirituality play an important part in the individual's/family's life?
- **Affiliation:** Does the individual/family identify with a formalized religion or spiritual community?
- **Culture:** How does the individual's/family's cultural background influence the way they think about life, death, health, or the way they care for themselves? How would the individual/family like the health care provider to address any spiritual issues with them?
- **Traditions:** What religious practices does the individual/family feel they need to observe to expedite/enhance the healing process?

Each question is relatively benign and brings up the subject without making a value judgment regarding the patient's participation in religious activities. The way a patient answers the first question can guide any subsequent questions. For instance, if religious faith or spirituality does not play a part in the individual's or family's life, there is no need to continue. If it does, or if the answer is equivocal, the provider can proceed to the next questions to find out more about the extent of their religious commitment.

An important factor to keep in mind throughout the interview is that many people encountered in the health care system are in a crisis situation. They may be angry at God, questioning their faith, or in some other way demonstrating a behavior or rhetoric that is not consistent with their actual belief system. Sorting through this may be difficult. If other family members or friends are available, they may be helpful in trying to put the pieces together so that the provider can ascertain the spiritual rubric that permeates the life of this person/family.

Using this or a similar approach will provide a framework within which health care providers can elicit a spiritual history from their patients. Having addressed the issue, it may be evident that most patients are very willing and perhaps even eager to discuss it further. After all, spirituality is important to many patients, whether it is important to the provider or not. Many want to discuss it, and who better to discuss it with than someone who is concerned for them not just physically but spiritually as well?

1

Perinatal Health Care Issues of African American Women

Cheryl Killion

In a country composed of a kaleidoscope of immigrants, the experience of African Americans* in the United States has no parallel. Although there is evidence that blacks arrived in the Americas from Africa well before the 17th century, most were forcibly brought to this country by Europeans and enslaved over the course of nearly 3 centuries.[1,2] The experience of slavery and the subsequent sequelae of segregation, discrimination, racism, and oppression have indelibly marked the daily experiences, family structure, and health of contemporary blacks.

Slavery brought 2 phenotypically and culturally distinct peoples together in a dominant-subordinate relationship so intertwined, complex, and ambivalent that it is impossible to describe the culture of one without reference to the other.[3] Although adaptations were bidirectional, deliberate attempts were made to eradicate African culture.[3,4] However, the Yoruba, Akan, Ibos, Angolans, and dozens of other groups among slaves forged their own life ways and became a single, although diverse, African American culture.[3] Drawing on deep African spiritual roots, these new Americans creatively transformed their languages, religion, art, music, and worldviews. They adapted family forms and family roles to compensate for their losses and to ensure their continuity. In accordance with their new environment, they altered the strategies they used to heal and stay well.[5] African American culture has been uniquely molded by historic, sociopolitical, and structural forces while

---

*African American, black American, and black will be used interchangeably.

1

simultaneously retaining elements of Africanism[5–7]; at the same time, it has continuously evolved into an integral component of the US mosaic.

Today the black population is estimated to be 34.6 million and constitutes 12.3% of the total population.[8] African Americans represent a heterogeneous population. Currently approximately 5% of the black population in the United States comprises foreign-born immigrants from Africa and the Caribbean.[9] Spanish-speaking immigrants of African descent from Central and South America also add to the mix.[9] Although the historic context of these groups differs from that of blacks born in the United States, the influence of slavery and/or colonialism of their ancestors also shaped their experiences and worldviews.[1,7] More recent immigrants of African descent often continue to identify with their home country as they become acclimated to American culture.[10] The heritage of many blacks also includes mixed ancestry of other ethnic/racial groups.[9]

Although most African Americans are Christians, with Protestantism predominating, blacks are also practicing members of the other major religions.[11] For example, black Americans are estimated to comprise approximately 24% of the Muslim (Orthodox Islam) population in the United States, the fastest-growing religion in the country.[12] In addition, a sizeable number of blacks are among the followers of Jehovah's Witnesses, a sect that has as one of its beliefs that it is a sin to accept blood transfusions.[13,14]

While African Americans are dispersed throughout the 50 states, most (87%) reside in urban areas; are concentrated in New York, Washington, DC, and 13 southern states[9]; and are more likely to live in racially segregated communities.[15] In 2000 there were 8.5 million black families, 44% of which were married-couple families.[8] More than half of all American blacks (approximately 17 million) are females. African American families are generally younger and larger than white American families, with an average family size of 3.5

people per household.[15] In the year 2020 nearly 1 out of 5 children of school age and 1 out of 6 adults of prime working age (25–59 years old) are projected to be African American.[16] Approximately 12% of African American children reside with a grandparent; 40% of these children have a grandparent as their primary caretaker.[15]

African Americans are represented in all socioeconomic groups. While some of the most influential positions in the United States are occupied by African Americans, blacks are also among the poorest, the most underemployed , and the least educated,[16] with 29% estimated to have incomes below the poverty line.[17] Inadequate income carries over into other spheres of daily life that affect health, including inadequate housing, malnutrition, the stress of constantly struggling to make ends meet, dangerous jobs, and little or no preventive health care[9]; furthermore, 80% of those among the lower socioeconomic strata are headed by women.[17] While more affluent African Americans may not have these identical issues, they regularly face obstacles related to their race that profoundly affect their quality of life and health. Gross inequities in the form of residential differentials, occupational discrimination, wealth inequalities, and interpersonal racism permeate the life experiences of all socioeconomic groups, despite phenomenal progress over the years.[18] Resilience, resistance, and the forging of social ties have enabled many African Americans to overcome some of these barriers.[10]

Health and Illness

African Americans do not have a monolithic approach to maintaining health, preventing disease, or coping with illness. Health beliefs and behaviors may be influenced by numerous factors: the person's socioeconomic status, urban versus rural residence, age, gender, or whether the individual is US or foreign born. The individual's expectations regarding the health care system are also important. Indeed, cross-cultural interactions between African American patients and health care providers may be marked by differences in understanding and communication, leading to mistrust and a lack of participation by blacks in their health care planning.[15,19,20] Additional cultural nuances of interpersonal interactions within the health care setting include issues of eye contact, facial expressions, touch, language, and symbolism that contribute to the patient's perceptions about insensitive or hasty, non-caring treatment.[15] An important demonstration of respect for the individual is the manner in which a patient is greeted; for example, it is considered respectful for health care providers to introduce themselves with a handshake and address patients as Mrs/Ms, rather than by their first names.

Evidence also shows that many of the core beliefs and self-care practices of blacks reflect, at least in part, the key tenets of a confluence of African philosophies. For example, among blacks, a representative pattern is a lifestyle of acquiescing to and synchronizing with nature rather than challenging it.[21] African Americans prefer the natural way and may exhibit an aversion for synthetically prepared medications or a reluctance to experience invasive procedures. Focus is on maintaining balance within the individual, between the individual and the environment, and with the cosmos. The body, mind, and environment must function in harmony for the individual to experience optimal health. Maintaining linkages with others in the community and with one's ancestors is critical and underscores the primacy of relationships. In fact, in many African traditions of healing, an understanding of social conflict and its impact may be pivotal for initiating the healing process.[22] The proximate cause or specific etiology is paramount, with germ theory, for instance, being useful only for explaining the medium through which health problems manifest themselves.[21]

The role of spirituality in maintaining wellness is strong within the African American community. As an extension of maintaining balance between the cosmos and the individual, many African Americans view maintaining health as a collaborative effort with God, whom they perceive to be the ultimate healer. When one's life is synchronous with

God's teachings, energy is derived that provides the strength to endure illness, accept inevitable death, or rejoice in a full recovery.[23] This personal relationship with God is manifested in and magnified by connectedness with one's extended family and a general sense of collectivism within the community. Importantly, illness is often perceived to be more of a state of mind than the condition of one's body.[24] The spiritual or religious experiences of African Americans shape their beliefs about the causes of illness, influence their treatment choices, and, for some individuals, promote a strong reliance on religious faith and prayer for healing or as an alternative to traditional medical care. This strong faith fosters a preference for life-sustaining procedures and medical care among some African Americans. For others, however, a sense of fatalism that views illness or death as "natural," unavoidable, or the "will of God" may influence their health care–seeking behaviors, responses to treatment options, or compliance with preventive health care recommendations.[15]

The full range of behaviors is evident among African Americans in their quest for health. Preventive measures are engaged in, particularly among those who have a number of options for nutrition, exercise, leisure activities, and health insurance. Others are less proactive and consider themselves to be "well" as long as they can go about their daily routines and can perform their usual tasks.[21] One interpretation of the often-quipped phrase "I'm blessed!" is that an individual can find something in his or her life for which to be grateful, no matter what their situation is. African American women, more often than men (or perhaps in a different manner than men), do not feel that they have the luxury of becoming ill. Moreover, illness is an affront to their well-being and may be perceived by some as a sign of weakness. Symptoms may be minimized, ignored, denied, or excused away because of multiple obligations and burdens of daily living that take priority over women taking care of their own needs.[25] After some self-diagnosing occurs, over-the-counter or home remedies may be tried.

Severity, frequency, and duration of symptoms, in conjunction with altered ability to perform regular activities, usually prompt women to seek formalized health care. Urgings from family members may also be a factor. Attitudes toward the health care system and past experiences with it circumscribe the personal perceptions of health and related health care–seeking behaviors.

High morbidity and mortality rates are a common reality in the African American community. African Americans have disproportionately more undetected diseases, as well as higher disease and illness rates from infectious conditions such as tuberculosis and sexually transmitted diseases including human immunodeficiency virus (HIV) and acquired immunodeficiency syndrome (AIDS); more chronic conditions such as hypertension and diabetes; and more potentially lethal diseases such as cancer, stroke, accidents, pneumonia, and shorter life expectancies than whites.[9] Human immunodeficiency virus and AIDS are the leading cause of death for African Americans between the ages of 25 and 44 years, with a death rate 9-fold higher for black women than white women.[15] The overall health status and disease patterns of the African Ameri-can population have been attributed to genetics, social environment, and lifestyles.

Tobacco, alcohol, and substance use are among the major risk factors that contribute to the burden of disease experienced by women and their children. Although smoking rates are lower among black than white adolescent girls, by age 35 to 44 years more than 35% of African American women smoke.[15] A similar usage pattern exists for alcohol as well, resulting in higher rates of fetal alcohol syndrome in the African American population. Although rates of illicit drug use are comparable for whites, Hispanics, and blacks during adolescence and early adulthood, by age 35 years documented rates for drug use among blacks exceeds that of whites or Hispanics. Among high school students, marijuana usage is similar across the 3 racial/ethnic groups, with Hispanic and white students reporting more likely usage of cocaine/crack, speed, heroin, or phencyclidine than black students.[15,26] Although substance use is common during pregnancy in all segments of the population, it is noteworthy that for illicit drug use, blacks are more likely to be tested and reported than their white counterparts. Moreover, involuntary foster care placement of newborns is mandated more frequently for blacks than for other groups.[27,28]

Biological, social, and genetic correlates of a number of disorders contribute to the higher incidences of substance abuse among African Americans, but it is difficult to disentangle the effects of each. Evidence suggests, however, that social disparities between African Americans and the general population have more influence over disease prevalence than genetic difference.[29] For example, access issues significantly affect the health status of blacks. African Americans are twice as likely as whites to be uninsured, are more likely to experience difficulties receiving appropriate and needed health care, have less choice where they receive care, have less access to regular sources of care, and report more negative experiences with the health care system.[9] These realities have influenced the use of African-based traditions, which affirm the heritage of African Americans and simultaneously are a response to circumstances of day-to-day existence. Because of past and current lack of access to health care services, discrimination, and racism encountered in health care facilities, many African Americans have developed alternative ways of interpreting and taking care of their needs.

Pregnancy/Prenatal Care

African Americans view pregnancy as a natural condition, although the increased vulnerability of the woman and the fetus during this time is readily acknowledged. Usually a cause for celebration, pregnancy symbolizes hope and continuity; for some, it is perceived to be the ultimate manifestation of womanhood and manhood. However, the positive experience of childbearing is marred all too often by illness or complications, which may result in death.

In 2000 the maternal mortality rate for African Americans was 20.3

per 100,000 live births from deliveries and complications of pregnancy, childbirth, and the puerperium,[30] 4-fold higher than the rate for white or Hispanic women. Disorders and conditions disproportionately affecting African American women that may have an impact on pregnancy include asthma, diabetes, uterine fibroids, hypertension (chronic and pregnancy-induced), lupus, sickle cell anemia, HIV, pelvic inflammatory disease (PID), and multiple births.[31] Black and Hispanic women account for 80% of HIV-infected women in the United States. The seroprevalence rates for HIV in pregnant women vary by country of origin (0%–0.6% in North America, 0.6% in Latin America, 2.4% in Caribbean countries, and 8.8% in Sub-Saharan Africa).[32] The implementation of prenatal prevention strategies, including HIV testing and counseling as well as antiretroviral therapy, including azidothymidine treatment of the pregnant woman with HIV infection and her newborn, has led to a 75% reduction in perinatal HIV transmission and a decline in the vertical transmission from 25% to 30% to 4% to 8%. Nevertheless, 62% of HIV-infected children in the United States are black.[33,34]

Infant mortality rates are twice as high among African Americans as those of the general population.[35] Low birth weight infants, due to prematurity and/or intrauterine growth restriction (small for gestational age babies), are born into African American families 3 times more than into white families.[30] These gaps have remained essentially unchanged over several decades despite significant improvements in perinatal care and survival. Reported disparities in infant mortality rates between black and white infants exist even when marital status, age, and in-come are similar,[36] and even among higher socioeconomic status, college-educated African American women.

The percentage of women entering prenatal care during the first trimester has increased steadily; however, a significant disparity between black and white women still exists, with 73% of African American women initiating prenatal care in the first trimester compared with 85% of white women. Even among those black women receiving first trimester prenatal care, only 67% are considered to be receiving adequate care.[37] Complications reported in 1998 during labor and delivery for black women occurred at a rate of 38 per 100 deliveries.[37]

Although inadequate prenatal care is frequently associated with poor outcomes, there are other factors that may explain the disproportionately high incidence of infant morbidity and mortality rates among black women. These include racial disparities in housing, exposure to environmental pollutants, low wages, inequities in employment, limited access to public facilities, and spacing intervals of less than 9 months between pregnancies.[38–40] In addition, generational effects are hypothesized to play an important role, such that a fetus develops in an intrauterine environment that bears the effects of its mother's own gestation, not just the current pregnancy state (Barker Hypothesis). In 2001 the mean birth weight for black infants was 3,135 g (6 lb 14 oz), 264 g (8.8 oz) less than white infants, whose mean birth weight was 3,399 g (7 lb 8 oz).

There is a tendency to focus solely on changing the lifestyles and daily habits of African Americans to promote more positive outcomes. For example, maintaining an adequate diet prior to, and during, the prenatal period is emphasized. Low income African Americans are often enrolled in the Special Supplemental Nutrition Program for Women, Infants, and Children (WIC) and receive food stamps.[40] While such programs have been beneficial, little consideration has been given to the fact that the nutritional status and dietary habits of African Americans have evolved from a unique cultural heritage, the remnants of which are inextricably enmeshed with their current daily life experiences.

Traditionally, African diets consisted of leafy, green vegetables; yams; okra; cassava; fresh fruits; seeds and nuts; and small amounts of meat, fish, and poultry.[41,42] On arriving in the Americas, however, the diet and culinary patterns of Africans were tempered by hardship, resulting in altered cooking methods, significant changes in the diet composition, and reliance on residual, leftover, and scrap foods. The cooking liquid from vegetables and meat was transformed into soups, stews, and gravies and often used for the dipping of biscuits or cornbread. Feasts were made from fatty and salty "throwaways" given to them for the main meals,[41,42] including chitterlings, ham hocks, pork rinds, pigs' feet, neck bones, and other components of what may be called "soul food."[43] Recent adaptations of these foods have found their way to the African American's table; for example, smoked turkey wings are sometimes substituted for ham hocks or fat backs for seasoning in greens and other dishes. Food preparation methods often include frying, excess salt use, and a tendency to overcook vegetables; meals tend to be large and heavy. Specific foods, flavors, food preparation practices, and meals may be used consciously or unconsciously, to preserve traditions, maintain group identity or solidarity, or for curative purposes.[44] In conjunction with high caloric intakes, 68% of black women reportedly do not regularly engage in exercise or physical activity.[15]

Contemporary African Americans continue to enjoy soul food as well as a wide range of cuisines; indeed, a growing number are vegetarians. Opportunities to appropriately counsel black women preconceptionally or during pregnancy may be missed if it is assumed that all eat one type of diet. Diets are consumed according to taste, nutritional value, availability, and affordability. For example, low-income families who reside in inner cities must rely on neighborhood, privately owned grocery stores (and sometimes convenience stores) for the bulk of their food because few of the major grocery store chains are located in these areas; thus the variety of food options available to them is limited and their prices are much higher.[45] Moreover, the privately owned grocers tend not to have an abundance of fresh fruit, vegetables, and meats. Fast foods and junk foods, thus, sometimes serve as convenient fillers.

Approximately 75% of African Americans are lactose intolerant; this fact has special implications for the childbearing family. Supplementary sources of vitamin D and calcium may need to be added to their diets, although lactose is usually digested readily by the newborn.[46] In addition, pica, an eating behavior that is manifested by a craving for oral ingestion of a given substance that is unusual in type and/or quantity, is fairly common among African American pregnant women[47]; substances that may be eaten are chalk, laundry starch, ice shavings, lead paint chips, and, most especially, clay (geophagia). Reports in the literature are conflicting regarding an association between women with pica and iron deficiency anemia, dysfunctional labor (caused by fecal impaction), and poor perinatal outcomes such as prematurity and low birth weight.[48,49] Unless specifically asked, expectant mothers are not likely to reveal that they engage in the dietary practice of pica.

Closely aligned with the dietary habits of African American women is their ingestion of a variety of herbal teas during pregnancy. Decades ago, granny midwives regularly prescribed herbal teas such as black haw-root tea (to prevent spontaneous abortion) and wild cherry bark teas to ease "body troubles."[50] A number of African American pregnant women continue to drink senna and goldenseal teas. Raspberry leaf tea has also been used for generations as a preventive for nausea and to strengthen and relax uterine muscles, making contractions easier to bear.[51]

Certain proscriptions have been passed down that relate to a black woman's activity during pregnancy. A common belief, for example, was that the fetus could be strangled by the umbilical cord if the mother stretched her arms over her head.[52] Another is that an infant might be "marked" with a blemish or birthmark or have an aversion or preference for something as a consequence of a mother's thoughts or actions.[52,53] Such beliefs have diminished as young women are introduced to their babies via ultrasound, are exposed to pregnancy and birth through the media, and/or receive childbirth education. Grandmothers, however, have a strong influence and often assert their views as to how the mother views, prepares, and cares for the baby.

Labor and Delivery

African American mothers acknowledge the beauty and transformative experience of birth as they prepare for and experience this event. Many read about childbearing; some enroll in childbirth preparation classes; and others rely on advice from their mothers, grandmothers, friends, and female relatives.[40,51] Women who have previously given birth often use that experience as a gauge for preparing for subsequent births. For a number of African American women, the primary focus is on ensuring that their home and finances are in order and that their partner is available for the new arrival. This type of readiness often takes precedence over the physical and emotional preparedness for the actual birthing event.

African American women may be accompanied to the hospital by their spouse, their partner, a female family member, a friend, or the entire family. The woman may be in advanced labor when she arrives at the hospital. This may be a conscious decision because of her greater sense of comfort at home or due to her anxiety over how she will be received and treated in the hospital. Because of the higher incidence of high-risk pregnancies among black women, birthing events may be offset by a barrage of invasive procedures and technologic interventions; thus childbirth is often treated as a medical crisis.[9,40] African American women may feel a degree of powerlessness because their control over the birth experience is often usurped. The effect of this birthing quagmire is far greater for them than mothers from the general population because it is a pattern that is repeated in so many other areas of their lives. Interactions with black women are often based on stereotypic assumptions about their socioeconomic status, educational background, lifestyle, morals, and sexuality. As they enter health care settings, they often gear up to defend their rights and human dignity.

No generalizations can be made about how African American women cope with labor. Many make every effort to experience all aspects of the birthing process as naturally as possible, relying on inner strength, centering, and/or prayer. Some are stoic and others freely express their discomfort.[40,51] Most are grateful for pain relief, but many use their own personal strategies, such as rocking, music, breathing techniques, massage, and other distractions and/or comfort measures. Low-income African American women, a disproportionate number of whom are recipients of public assistance, are not readily offered epidurals for pain relief because Medicaid reimbursement for epidurals is significantly less than private insurance rates.[54–56] Thus some may have to endure pain, be heavily medicated, or receive general anesthesia for Cesarean births.

Postpartum and Newborn Care

Traditionally a pregnant black woman was believed to be in a physically and spiritually precarious state: a state of intense susceptibility to the outside as her body opened to and accommodated the fetus.[40] The period immediately following birth was a time of closure and restoration when boundaries between the inside and the outside were re-established. The postpartum period offered the infant a period of acclimatization after having been enclosed in the womb.[40] Thus the delivery and disposal of the placenta marked the end of one phase and the beginning of another. Some of these beliefs persist today and are reflected in postpartum measures that are taken to protect the body on the one hand and restrict it on the other. Women are to be shielded from drafts or wind. Pores, veins, and other parts of the body are usually thought to be closed systems that have been opened up in childbirth. As a precaution, some African American women continue to avoid washing their hair or taking tub baths during this time. The period after childbirth has also been viewed as a time for women to rid themselves of impurities.[53] A number of herbal teas may be used. Sassafras tea may be taken to cleanse the blood. Castor oil mixed with lemon juice is still sometimes ingested to purge or clean out one's "system" after childbirth.[51] Another means of purging is regular douching once menstruation resumes and/or after sexual intercourse; this practice has been associated with PID, ectopic pregnancy, infertility, and cervical cancer.[57]

With obesity becoming almost epidemic among children and adolescents, many African American women are entering pregnancy with excessive weight. In addition, factors such as higher parity, low rates of breastfeeding, low activity levels, and several medical conditions, including diabetes, hypertension, and osteoarthritis, increase their tendency to gain and retain weight after giving birth[58] and make the challenge of maintaining a balance between rest and physical activities and exercise even greater.[59] The resumption of a woman's other responsibilities, such as the need to return to work, care for the newborn and other children, and lack of access to fitness facilities, equipment, and organized groups, further prevent many African American women from actively and consistently engaging in physical fitness activities after giving birth.[58] Despite this population's high rate of obesity, African American women tend to have positive body images, and less stigma is associated with being overweight. Thus health promotional strategies that are centered on the significance of weight loss to improving one's health status are the most effective.

The naming of the newborn has special significance among African Americans. It provides an opportunity to exercise control over one's identity, honor one's ancestors, and provide continuity with, and establish pride in, one's heritage.[60] During slavery, names were points of contention and conflict between slave owner and slave. The practice of dual naming was common. While the given name of a newborn was often disregarded and the slave owner renamed the infant, slave family members and friends used the original or "basket" name in close circles. In addition, slave families had to take on the surname of their owner, at least until emancipation.[61] Traditional practices of naming infants according to conditions surrounding the birth, a particular current or past situation, appearance or temperament of the child, or the attitude of the parent toward the birth still exist today. For example, African kinship relations were preserved by naming sons after fathers who were often forcibly separated from the family.[62] Frequently an infant was named after a grandparent or great aunt or uncle. Evidence exists of the necronymic practice of naming the child after a dead sibling. Often the naming of an infant was delayed to ensure that the baby lived.[62]

Nicknaming was, and continues to be, very widespread among African Americans. Not only are nicknames endearing, they provided the slaves with some degree of control and continue to allow for the retention of African patterns.[63] During the 1960s proponents of the Black Nationalist movement urged black Americans to reclaim their African roots by adopting African names.[64] Contemporary African Americans have reinstituted the practice of having a naming ceremony to celebrate the birth of their newborn.[65] Because of historic and current events, African Americans give their newborns names that are distinct in their meaning, pronunciation, and spelling.

In 2001 72.7% of white women breastfed their newborns immediately following birth compared with 52.9% of African American women; at 6 months of age, only 21.9% of black women were still breastfeeding their infants while almost twice as many white women were continuing to do so.[66] These racial differences represent almost a complete reversal from the previous century. During the early 1800s wet nursing was common as numerous black slaves nursed white infants as well as their own.[67] Breastfeeding continued as the primary mode of infant feeding for black women up through the 1950s, at which time breastfeeding among all women declined rapidly. However, having been raised to consciousness by the feminist movement, many educated, middle class white women began to choose natural child-birth and quickly embraced nursing as part of the shift toward natura-listic health and healing. Conversely, most African American women, perhaps influenced by their alienation and isolation from the feminist movement, targeted by formula companies, and affected by work sche-dules, did not return to breastfeeding to the same degree. Thus by the mid-1960s, for the first time in American history, white women were more likely to breastfeed than black women.[68] Today women least like-ly to breastfeed are black, single, and residents of the South. Black women most likely to breastfeed match their white counterparts in that they tend to be older, college educated, and married.[68]

Many black women are reluctant to breastfeed their infants because of embarrassment; modesty; shame (feelings heightened by the socie-tal view of breasts as sex objects); irregular work hours; lack of sup-port in the job/school settings; the perceived loss of freedom; a lack of support from their partners; concern about their figures; a lack of ade-quate and accurate information about breastfeeding; a lack of support from health care providers, family, and/or friends; and limited or no postpartum assistance.[67–69]

African American women have adopted a number of ways of feed-ing their infants based on trial and error, their family's financial situa-tion, and assumptions about infants' physiologic nature, growth and development, nutritional needs, and the consistency of milk.[67,68] For example, they commonly give water to their newborn in addition to breastfeeding or formula feeding.[68] Some mothers readily com-bine formula feeding and breastfeeding while others mix cereal with formula in the bottle for infants when they are a few weeks old. Also, solid foods may be introduced earlier than the recommended schedule.[70]

African American mothers (and grandmothers) are diligent about cleanliness, hygiene, and other aspects of newborn care. Generous amounts of baby oil or petroleum jelly may be used to keep the skin well lubricated and the hair shiny. Newborn infants are often over-swaddled to keep the air away or to prevent the development of respiratory problems. Despite the general reduction in the incidence of sudden infant death syndrome (SIDS) for all populations, the incidence remains higher in the black population,[71] with African American infants twice as likely to die from SIDS than white infants. This may be because the significance of positioning infants for sleep and other factors related to the prevention of SIDS has not reached as many black families as needed. Indeed, concerns about the baby's comfort as well as fear of infants choking while on their backs make some mothers and grandmothers reluctant to place their babies on their backs or sides while in their cribs.

Family Planning

Compared with a national rate of 60% of all pregnancies being unintended, 70% of pregnancies in black women are unplanned.[72] Beliefs about normal body functions (ie, what constitutes normal menstrual flow), concern about their ability to conceive, and fear of untoward side effects of certain contraceptives often guide African Americans in their choices related to family planning.[73] Currently, most black women use oral contraceptives as their primary mode of family planning.[74] The use (or avoidance) of family planning services is often influenced by concerns about privacy, embarrassment about sexuality issues, and limited access and knowledge about specific contraceptive methods.[26] Beyond these factors, contraception conjures up a myriad of conflicting, contradictory, controversial, and confounding issues for African Americans that women in the general population do not have to face. For example, a perceived racist denigration of black childbearing, including deliberate campaigns to limit black fertility, is further complicated by sexist and religious norms within and outside of the black community.[75]

For African American women, birth control has always conjured up conflicts related to oppression versus liberation. During the eugenics movement, Margaret Sanger and others called for birth control programs to regulate the poor, immigrants, and blacks, based on theories of purported genetic inferiority. Some blacks of the period responded by opposing birth control as a form of "racial suicide or genocide" while others viewed contraception as a means of improving their health, the quality of their lives, and their life choices.[75,76]

During the 1960s and 1970s, thousands of poor, and disproportionately black, women were coercively sterilized under federally funded programs.[75] Women were threatened with termination of welfare benefits or denial of medical care if they did not consent to the procedure. An underlying assumption remains to this day that women who receive public assistance have children to obtain increased benefits, although no studies support this assumption.[77] More recently the debate about race and birth control has resurfaced, as poor black women have been encouraged to use long-lasting contraceptives such as hormonal implants and injectables.[75] Norplant was deemed to be a "solution to inner-city poverty" and predominantly black high schools were targeted for the introduction of this long-term contraceptive.[78,79] Family planning strategies for contemporary African Americans must involve advocating for women's freedom to use contraceptives while opposing abusive birth control practices.

Abortion has long been viewed with disapproval throughout the African American community. However, elective termination of pregnancy is perceived to be a necessary option in some circumstances and is contingent on one's religious beliefs.[10]

Bioethical Dilemmas

The recent proliferation of reproductive technologies has revolutionized childbearing. In particular, the scope of prenatal testing has widened to prenatal diagnosis, which can be perplexing, particularly in the event that a genetic defect is detected or the severity of fetal illness is determined. There is some evidence that African American women (and Latinas) are less likely to undergo prenatal diagnosis than white and Asian women.[80]

Despite the best intentions of health professionals to be neutral and to respect patients' preferences, the way in which information and available options are presented may be subject to subtle manipulation and bias.[81] In addition to the manner in which women and their families are counseled, a host of other factors have an effect on decision making: religious/spiritual orientation, reproductive history, family considerations and relationships, institutional policies, views about the pregnancy, timing, perceptions of and knowledge about the tests, and a myriad of other factors. Seeking spiritual guidance is a vital step for many parents as they ponder their options. Some denominations allow for prenatal diagnosis and pregnancy interruption whereas others are vehemently against any action taken if the tests reveal a problem. Some parents are reluctant to approach clergy, particularly if they anticipate that their decision may counter that of church doctrine. Others may refuse the tests because they believe that the outcome of the pregnancy represents God's will. They rely on God's guidance to help them care for and raise a child, regardless of the child's health status. Whatever the outcome, the child is viewed as a blessing. In addition to there being a religious or spiritual dilemma, a cultural issue exists as well.[74] A pregnant woman is a bearer of her heritage and a carrier of a legacy that is to be passed from generation to generation. The prospect of altering that opportunity may be overwhelming. African American women may be reluctant to undergo chorionic villi sampling or amniocentesis because they fear that such tests could harm the fetus or precipitate a miscarriage.

The family and the African American community are pivotal in providing the context for decision making; thus a family-centered approach is useful in seeking the involvement of those who are significant to expectant mothers.[82] Many black women are suspicious of some screening and diagnostic tests. Their distrust may be rooted in the long history of experimentation, mutilation, and negative treatment of blacks by the health care system.[83] The Tuskegee Syphilis Study, conducted from the 1930s to the 1960s, is still fresh in the minds of many.[84] During the study, poor black men with syphilis were followed (without treatment) until they died to determine the "natural" history of the disease. In addition, procedures performed unnecessarily, such as unwarranted hysterectomies, haunt the individual and collective memories of many African Americans.[83] Thus the context and manner in which informed consent is broached is a particularly sensitive area. Technology has become so powerful in medicine that choices patients and families face "do not arise from the patients' worlds of experience but rather are created for them by institutional directives, the culture of hospitals, and the technological imperative."[74]

The provider-patient relationship is governed by the principles of *autonomy,* respect for a person's right to live by her or his own values, and *beneficence,* a health care professional's obligation to promote his or her patient's well-being. These 2 principles can come into conflict in the process of caring for a pregnant patient. Although competent, informed patients may refuse treatment choices, even if such decisions are life-threatening or lead to a patient's death, pregnancy is one circumstance in which the interests of the fetus must be considered in addition to the rights of the expectant mother.[85] Thus the beneficence obligations of the health care provider to the child require that potentially life-sustaining treatments, including blood product transfusions, be administered where appropriate. This is based on the doctrine of *parens patriae,* the authority of the state to preserve the lives of minors.[85] Given the higher complication rates and mortality for African American women, it is critical to discuss with each patient her faith-based beliefs and discuss available options. If the birth of a low birth weight or premature baby, or an infant with a hemolytic anemia, major birth defect, or serious illness is anticipated, it is equally important to discuss with the family the available treatment choices for minimizing and managing blood loss, anemia, and the potential need for administration of blood products. In the case of black families who are devout Jehovah's Witnesses, it may be necessary to obtain a court order mandating the needed blood products.[86]

Death/Burial Rites

"I believe that on some deeper level Black women are used to tragedy.... Death is not a stranger to our lives, to our world. We've lost our fathers to heart attacks, our brothers to frontline battles, our husbands and lovers to black-on-black crime, or police brutality.... All this while grappling with dehumanizing conditions...the slow but steady death of our people...."[87]

Death and loss are part of the daily reality of many African Americans. Perinatal loss is devastating to families, especially because so much hope is associated with birth. No parent is adequately prepared for this type of event. Regardless of the gestational timing of the loss, the grieving response is usually intense. When an early pregnancy loss occurs, however, women are not expected to grieve and often do not receive the support they need. Their experience is often minimized and treated as inconsequential. Because pregnancy and infant loss is fairly common among African Americans, their experiences may even be "normalized."[88] The perception that black women are "superstrong" and can handle anything may be inadvertently imposed without exploring the woman's reaction and acknowledging the full impact of her loss.[25,88]

While grieving responses of all women who experience perinatal loss vary, healing strategies of one group of African American women included finding purpose or meaning for their loss, responding to an inner voice guiding them to specific actions to begin healing themselves, drawing from their religion or spirituality, finding comfort in knowing that their infant was "in a better place" (ancestors were caring for their infants), and compartmentalizing their grief to alleviate emotional pain. The mothers used a variety of strategies to maintain some connection with the deceased infant while simultaneously attempting to move on with their lives.[88]

A striking commonality within the African American is that peri-natal loss may have occurred in previous generations, opening old wounds for grandmothers when their daughters experience the death of an infant (R. Husband, oral communication, 2000). The reality of the black experience, having been circumscribed by persistent injustices and disproportionate morbidity yet sustained protests and strides, sets the backdrop against which rituals of grieving become a mechanism for support and survival.[89] While beliefs about death and related rituals are based primarily on the religious inclinations of the parents, some degree of cultural specificity is evident as well.

Funerals are a vehicle for expressing the rituals of death and reflect a belief in life after death. For deceased black infants, a family visitation period and viewing is generally followed by a graveside burial. However, "full blown" funerals have been conducted with a church service, including a eulogy, scripture, and music on behalf of the dead baby. The obituary, although necessarily short, may include the baby's first photograph. Recounts of personal remembrances and expressions of the baby's special qualities, such as the way the baby smiled, cried, or even moved in utero, are included in the document as well as in the eulogy. It is common for families to place a stuffed animal, a rattle, or some other personal item of the infant in the casket. Babies have been buried wearing the bib they often wore during feedings. Some parents take photographs of their baby in the coffin and may clip a braid or lock of the baby's hair to keep (R. Husband, oral communication, 2000). The grave site may be decorated with flowers. Sometimes personal items of the baby are placed on the grave and, on occasion, a feeding has been left for the deceased infant to consume (R. Husband, oral communication, 2000). In some parts of the rural south, the African practice of placing broken pieces of pottery or earthenware on the grave is still practiced. This ritual symbolizes not only the destruction of the body by death, but also the last strength of the deceased person as contained in the last object that may have been used on his or her behalf.[90] As with the funeral of an adult, a family meal is usually planned after the service, although this is left to the discretion of the parents.

Mortuary rituals are an opportunity for expressing the symbolic ideals of African Americans. The ideals are reflected in giving a unique, often elaborate, "home-going" to celebrate the brief life of a hoped-for child. Thus dignity is created at death often to disguise the "social death" that may have occurred in everyday life.[89,90]

Every African American Woman Is Unique

African Americans are a heterogeneous people, diverse in physical appearance, lifestyles, and beliefs; yet, they hold in common the legacy of slavery. This experience continues to have a strong impact on the quality of life and health of African Americans, regardless of their socioeconomic status. Giving birth is a natural event over which African American women seek more control. They desire the same access and quality of care afforded to women in the general population without being labeled and treated as if they are medical problems. In this chapter, specific and contextual information was provided that hopefully will foster a desire to learn more about a grossly misunderstood people. It is by no means an exhaustive overview nor does it provide a recipe for health professionals.

Perinatal Health Care Issues of African American Women: Key Highlights

Demographic/Psychosocial/Spiritual Characteristics

- Blacks are estimated at 34.6 million (12.3%) of the total US population.
- African Americans are a heterogeneous population.
- Approximately 5% of the black population in the United States are immigrants from Africa and the Caribbean.
- Blacks are dispersed throughout the 50 states; 87% reside in urban

areas and are concentrated in New York; Washington, DC; and 13 southern states.

- African Americans are strong, creative, and resilient and strive for optimal health.
- Blacks derive much support from their extended families, including ancestors.
- Blacks have developed alternative ways of taking care of their needs, based on their African heritage as well as past and current experiences with health care access.
- Blacks enter the health care system with a polite yet vigilant demeanor.
- For many African Americans, there is an inherent distrust of the health care system, less satisfaction with the provider-patient relationship, and a perception that health care providers are not as attentive or interested in their health care needs.

Prenatal Care
- Pregnancy is viewed as a natural state; thus prenatal care may be delayed.
- Prenatal care may not be readily sought because of negative experiences with the health care system.
- Life circumstances may challenge the ability of low-income African American women to seek prenatal care or keep appointments.

Prenatal Testing
- Screening for sickle cell anemia is essential.
- African American women vary in their reaction to results of prenatal screening such as amniocentesis and chorionic villi sampling.
- Higher rates of pregnancy complications and maternal mortality require optimal health surveillance and prenatal screening.

Pregnancy Diet
- Adequacy of diet may be dependent on availability and affordability of healthy food.
- The diet of African Americans consists of a wide range of foods and may include foods that are high in salt, fat, and carbohydrates.
- Lactose intolerance is common, often resulting in associated insufficient dietary intakes of calcium and vitamin D.
- Pica is common among pregnant, low-income African American women.
- A variety of herbal teas may be taken for nausea and other pregnancy-related conditions.

Pregnancy-Related Beliefs/Taboos
- Conflicts are avoided to ensure positive outcomes.
- Preoccupations of the mother may "mark" the baby.
- Reproductive events may be predicted by the position of the moon.

Labor and Delivery
- The designated partner in labor is usually the father of the child or a female family member or friend.
- African American women prefer female attendants, but are more concerned about the proficiency and sensitivity of the professional.
- Reactions to labor vary.
- Low-income African American women may not have the same options for pain relief as other women.

Postpartum Care
- The postpartum period is a critical part of the birthing process for restoring women's health.
- Restfulness is as important as exercise, although both may be difficult to achieve.

Postpartum Diet
- No particular diets are prescribed.
- Special teas may be taken to cleanse the body of impurities.

Neonatal Care
- Cleanliness and appropriate feeding are the focus of newborn care.
- Naming the infant has special significance.
- Rates of SIDS remain twice as high for black infants.

Breastfeeding/Breast Care
- Although breastfeeding initiation and continuation rates among African American women have increased significantly, they remain below Healthy People 2010 objectives.
- African American women who breastfeed tend not to initiate and sustain exclusive breastfeeding through 6 months postpartum.
- Reasons given for not breastfeeding relate to problems with self-image, fear or pain, perceived inadequate milk supply, the competing needs of family and work, and limited assistance and support.

Family Planning
- Oral contraceptives are the most commonly used form of birth control.
- Although condoms are used with regularity, other barrier methods have low usage.
- Family planning has been mired by tension between freedom of choice and abusive birth control practices.

Family Involvement
- The husband or male partner, and/or mother or female relative, are involved throughout the childbearing experience, but the entire family, including extended kin, may be present for the birth.
- The maternal grandmother plays a significant role, particularly during pregnancy and the postpartum period.

Religious Practices
- Within the first few months after birth, the newborn is either christened or blessed.
- God is viewed as the ultimate healer.

- Prayer is a vital healing strategy.
- African Americans are primarily Protestants; they are also followers of all the other major religions.

Pregnancy Termination/Miscarriage
- Elective termination of pregnancy is perceived to be a necessary option in some circumstances and is contingent on the African American's religious beliefs.

Bioethical Dilemmas
- Perinatal diagnosis and the potential for fetal intervention and/or neonatal treatment have become more routine, creating perplexing dilemmas for prospective parents.
- Decision making is influenced by religious factors, reproductive history, family considerations, timing of tests, institutional relationships, views about the pregnancy, perceptions of knowledge about the tests, and trust in the health care system and its providers.

Death/Burial Rites
- Premature death in the African American community is a common occurrence.
- Perinatal loss may have occurred in previous generations, opening old wounds for grandmothers when their daughters experience the death of an infant.
- Life after death is a core belief and is reflected in death rituals.
- Burial rituals are dependent on the religious affiliation and inclinations of the parents.
- Burial rites reflect giving dignity when this aspect was not necessarily given to families during life.

References

1. Torres A, Whitten NE. General introduction: to forge the future in the fires of the past. An interpretative essay on racism, domination, resistances, and liberations. In: Torres A, Whitten N, eds. *Blackness in Latin America and the Caribbean.* Bloomington, IN: Indiana University Press; 1998:3–34

2. Eltis D. *The Rise of African Slavery in the Americas.* Cambridge, MA: Cambridge University Press; 2000

3. Feagin JR, Feagin CB. *Racial and Ethnic Relations.* Upper Saddle River, NJ: Prentice-Hall, Inc.; 1996

4. Genovese ED. *Roll Jordan, Roll: The World the Slaves Made.* New York, NY: Vintage Books; 1972

5. Levine LW. *Black Culture and Black Consciousness.* Oxford, UK: Oxford University Press; 1977

6. Airhihenbuwa CD. Cultural identity and healthy lifestyles among African Americans: a new direction for health interventions. *Ethnicity Dis.* 2000;10:148–164

7. Holloway JE. The origins of African-American culture. In: Holloway JE, ed. *Africanisms in American Culture.* Bloomington, IN: Indiana University Press; 1990:1–18

8. McKinnon J. The black population in the United States: March 2002 population characteristics. In: *Current Population Reports.* Washington, DC: Bureau of the Census, US Department of Commerce; April 2003

9. National Institutes of Health. Factors affecting the health of women of color: black Americans. In: *Women of Color Health Data Book.* Bethesda, MD: Office of the Director, National Institutes of Health; 1997:12–16

10. Billingsley A. *Climbing Jacob's Ladder: The Enduring Legacy of African American Families.* New York, NY: Simon & Schuster; 1992

11. Taylor RJ, Chatters LM. Religious life. In: Jackson JS, ed. *Life in Black America.* Thousand Oaks, CA: Sage Publications; 1991:105–123

12. Turner RT. *Islam in the African American Experience.* Bloomington, IN: Indiana University Press; 1997

13. Kosmin B, Lachman S. *One Nation Under God.* New York, NY: Harmony Books; 1993

14. Muramoto O. Recent developments in the medical care of Jehovah's Witnesses. *West J Med.* 1999;170:297–301

15. Kaiser Permanente National Diversity Council. *A Provider's Handbook on Culturally Competent Care: African Americans*. Oakland, CA: The Kaiser Permanent Institute for Culturally Competent Care; 1999

16. Hopp SW, Herring P. Promoting health among black American populations: an overview. In: Huff RM, Kline MV, eds. *Promoting Health in Multicultural Populations*. Thousand Oaks, CA: Sage Publications; 1999:201–221

17. US Census Bureau. *Persons Below Poverty Level and Below 125 Percent of Poverty Level: Statistical Abstract of the United States: 2000*. Washington, DC: US Census Bureau; 2002

18. Pattillo-McCoy M. Middle class, yet black: a review. *Afr Am Res Perspect.* 2001;5:25–37

19. Doescher MP, Saver BG, Franks P, Fiscella K. Racial and ethnic disparities in perceptions of physician style and trust. *Arch Fam Med.* 2000;9:1156–1163

20. Cooper-Patrick L, Gallo JJ, Gonzales JJ, et al. Race, gender, and partnership in the patient-physician relationship. *JAMA.* 1999;282:583–589

21. Airhihenbuwa CO. *Health and Culture: Beyond the Western Paradigm.* Thousand Oaks, CA: Sage Publications; 1995:25–62, 87–106

22. Feierman S, Janzen JM. Introduction. In: Feierman S, Janzen JM, eds. *The Social Bases of Health and Healing in Africa.* Berkeley, CA: University of California Press; 1992:1–23

23. Abrums M. "Jesus will fix it after awhile." Meanings and health. *Soc Sci Med.* 2000;50:89–105

24. Watson W. Introduction. In: Watson W, ed. *Black Folk Medicine.* New Brunswick, NJ: Transaction Publishers; 1984

25. Collins PH. *Black Feminist Thought.* New York, NY: Routledge; 2000

26. Grunbaum JA, Kann L, Kinchen SA, et al. Youth risk behavior surveillance— United States, 2001. *J Sch Health.* 2002;72:313–328. Available at http://www.cdc.gov/nccdphp/dash/yrbs. Accessed July 15, 2003

27. Chasnoff IJ. The prevalence of illicit-drug or alcohol use during pregnancy and discrepancies in mandatory reporting in Pinellas County, Florida. *N Engl J Med.* 1990;322:1202–1206

28. Neuspiel DR, Zingman TM, Templeton VH, DiStabile P, Drucker E. Custody of cocaine-exposed newborns: determinants of discharge decisions. *Am J Public Health.* 1993;83:1726–1729

29. Williams DR, Yu Y, Jackson JS. Racial difference in physical and mental health. *J Health Psych.* 1997;2:335–351

30. US Census Bureau. Infant, maternal and neonatal mortality rates and fetal mortality ratios by race: 1980 to 1998. *Statistical Abstract of the United States: 2000.* Available at http://www.census.gov/prod/200/pubs/ statab/sec02.pdf. Accessed July 14, 2003

31. York R, Tulman L, Brown K. Postnatal care in low-income urban African American women: relationships to level of prenatal care sought. *J Perinatol.* 2000;1:34–40

32. World Health Organization. *AIDS Epidemic Update.* Geneva, Switzerland: Joint United Nations Programme on HIV/AIDS; 2002. Available at: http://www.unaids.org. Accessed February 15, 2003

33. Centers for Disease Control and Prevention. *Status of Perinatal HIV Prevention: US Declines Continue.* Atlanta, GA: Centers for Disease Control and Prevention; 1999. Available at http://www.cdc.gov/hiv/ pubs/facts/perinatl.htm. Accessed July 15, 2003

34. Maldonado M. State of emergency: HIV/AIDS among African Americans. *Body Posit.* 1999;12:32–35

35. Centers for Disease Control and Prevention. Infant mortality and low birth weight among black and white infants. United States, 1980–2000. *MMWR Morb Mortal Wkly Rep.* 2002;51:589–592

36. Schoendorf KC, Hoque CJ, Kleinman JC, Ravley D. Mortality among infants of blacks as compared to white college educated parents. *N Engl J Med.* 1992;326:1522:15–56

37. US Department of Health and Human Services. *Healthy People 2010.* 2nd ed. Washington, DC: US Government Printing Office; 2000

38. Rutter DR, Quine L. Inequalities in pregnancy outcomes: a review of psychosocial and behavioral mediators. *Soc Sci Med.* 1990;30:553–568

39. Blackmore-Prince C, Iyasu S, Kendrick JS, et al. Are interpregnancy intervals between consecutive live births among black women associated with infant birth weight? *Ethnicity Dis.* 2000;10:106–112

40. Fraser GT. *African American Midwifery in the South: Dialogues of Birth, Race, and Memory.* Cambridge, MA: Harvard University Press; 1998

41. Harris JB. Celebrating our cuisine. In: White E, ed. *The Black Woman's Health Book: Speaking for Ourselves.* Seattle, WA: Seal Press; 1994;305–309

42. Lukes A, Cooper RS, Prewitt TE, Adeyeno AA, Forrester TE. Nutritional consequences of the African Diaspora. *Ann Rev Nutr.* 2001;21:47–71

43. Whitehead TL. In search of soul food and meaning: culture, food and health. In: Baer HA, Jones Y, eds. *African Americans in the South.* Athens, GA: University of Georgia Press; 1992:94–109

44. Airhihenbuwa CO, Kumanyika S. Cultural aspects of African American eating patterns. *Ethnicity Health.* 1996;1:245–261

45. Killion CM. Special health care needs of homeless pregnant women. *Adv Nurs Sci.* 1995;18:44–56

46. Sherwen LN, Scolovens MA, Weingarten CT. Nursing care of the childbearing family. Norwalk, CT: Appleton & Lange; 1991

47. Moore MC. Maternal and fetal nutrition. In: Lowdermilk PM, Perry SE, Bobak IM, eds. *Maternity and Women's Health Care.* St Louis: Mosby; 1977:169

48. Reid RM. Cultural and medical perspectives on geophagia. *Med Anthropol.* 1992;13:337–351

49. Lacey EP. Broadening the perspectives of pica. Literature review. *Public Health Rep.* 1990;105:29–35

50. Campbell M. *Folks Do Get Born.* New York, NY: Rinehardt; 1946

51. Brown D, Toussaint PA. *Mama's Little Baby: The Black Woman's Guide to Pregnancy, Childbirth, and the Baby's First Year.* New York, NY: Penguin Books; 1997

52. Frankel B. *Childbirth in the Ghetto: Folk Beliefs of Negro Women in a North Philadelphia Hospital Ward.* San Francisco, CA: Rason; 1977

53. Snow L. Traditional health beliefs and practices among lower class black Americans. *West J Med.* 1983;134:820–824

54. Bell ED, Penning DH, Cousineau EF, et al. How much labor is in a labor epidural? Manpower cost and reimbursement for an obstetric analogies service in a teaching institution. *Anesthesia.* 2000;92:851–858

55. Chestnut DH. How do we measure (the cost of) pain relief? *Anesthesia.* 2000;92:643

56. Obst IE, Nauenberg E, Buck GM. Maternal health insurance coverage as a determinant of obstetrical anesthesia care. *J Health Care Poor Underserved.* 2000;12:180

57. Aral SO, Mosher WD, Cates W. Vaginal douching among women of reproductive age in the United States 1988. *Am J Public Health.* 1992;82:210–214

58. Kumanyika S, Wilson JF, Guilford-Davenport M. Weight-related attitudes and behaviors of black women. *J Am Diet Assoc.* 1993;93:416–422

59. Sampselle CM, Seng J, Yeo J, Killion C, Oakley D. Physical activity and postpartum well-being. *J Obstet Gynecol Neonatal Nurs.* 1999;28:41–44

60. Cooke M. Naming, being, and black experiences. *Yale Rev.* 1978;68:167–186

61. Gates HL. *The Classic Slave Narrative.* New York, NY: Signet; 1897

62. Foster H. African patterns in the Afro-American family. *J Black Studies.*
    1983;14:201–232
63. Eklof B. *For Every Season: The Complete Guide to African Americans
    Celebrations: Traditional to Contemporary.* New York: HarperCollins;
    1997
64. Adeleke T. Black Americans, Africa and history: a reassessment of the
    Pan-African and identity paradigms. *West J Black Study.*1998;22:182–194
65. Hutcherson H. *Having Your Baby: A Guide for African American Women.*
    New York, NY: Ballatine Press; 1997
66. Ryan AS, Wenjun Z, Acosta A. Breastfeeding continues to increase into the
    new millennium. *Pediatrics.* 2002;110:1103–1109
67. Gardner J. The magic of mothers milk: breastfeeding your baby. In: White
    E, ed. *The Black Women's Health Book: Speaking for Ourselves.* Seattle, WA:
    Seal Press; 1994:310–318
68. Fooadi MA. Comparison of perspectives on breastfeeding between
    two generations of black American women. *J Am Acad Nurs Pract.*
    2001;13:34–38
69. Underwood S, Pridam K, Brwon L, et al. Infant feeding practices of
    low-income African American women in a central city community.
    J Com Health Nurs. 1997;14:189–205
70. Bronner Y, Gross SM, Caulfield L, et al. Early introduction of solid food
    among urban African-American participants in WIC. *J Am Diet Assoc.*
    1999;99:457–461
71. Adams EJ, Chavez, GF, Steen D, Shah R, Iyasu S, Krousett F. Changes in the
    epidemiologic profile of sudden infant death syndrome as rates decline
    among California infants: 1994–1995. *Pediatrics.* 1998;102:1445–1451
72. Roberts D. The pill at 40 — A new look at a familiar method: black
    women and the pill. *Fam Plann Perspest.* 2000;32:93–94
73. Killion C. Poverty and procreation among women: an anthropologic
    study with implications for health care providers. *J Nurse Midwife.*
    1998;43:273–278
74. US Census Bureau. *Race and Hispanic Origin Population Density of
    the United States: Use of Contraception.* Washington, DC: US Census
    Bureau; 1990
75. Roberts D. Black women and the pill. *Fam Plan Prospect.* 2000:32:92–93
76. Darity WA, Turner CB. Family planning, race consciousness and fear of
    race genocide. *Am J Public Health.* 1972;62:1454–1459

77. Wise P, Chavkin W, Romero D. Assessing the effects of welfare policies in reproductive and infant health. *Am J Public Health.* 1999;89:1514–1521

78. Litvan LM. Norplant program assailed; poor black girls seen as targets. *Washington Times.* December 4, 1992

79. Kimelan D. Poverty and Norplant: can contraception reduce the under class? *Philadelphia Inquirer.* December 12, 1990

80. Kuppermann M, Gates E, Washington AE. Racial ethnic difference in prenatal diagnostic test use and outcomes: preference, socioeconomic status, or patient knowledge. *Obstet Gynecol.* 1996;87:675–682

81. Kristol E. Picture perfect: the politics of prenatal testing. *First Things.* 1993;32:17–24

82. Galvin E, Boyers L, Schwartz PK, et al. Challenging the precepts of family centered care: testing of philosophy. *Pediatr Nurs.* 2000;26:625–633

83. Rapp R. Refusing prenatal diagnosis: the meanings of bioscience in a multicultural world. *Sci Technol Human Values.* 1998;23:45–70

84. Freimuth VS, Quinn SC, Thomas SB, Cole G, Zook E, Duncan T. African Americans' views on research and the Tuskegee Syphilis Study. *Social Sci Med.* 2001;52:797–808

85. Lewis JA. Genetics in perinatal nursing: clinical applications and policy considerations. *J Obstet Gynecol Neonat Nurs.* 2002;31:188–192

86. Schonholz DH. Blood transfusion and the pregnant Jehovah's Witness patient: avoiding a dilemma. *Mount Sinai J Med.* 1999;66:277–279

87. Davis BM. Speaking of grief: today I feel real low, I hope you understand. In: White E, ed. *The Black Women's Health Book: Speaking for Ourselves.* Seattle, WA: Seal Press; 1994:219–225

88. Van P. Breaking the silence of African American women: healing after pregnancy loss. *Health Care Women Int.* 2001:22:229–243

89. Secundy MC. Introduction: loss and grief. In: Secundy MC, ed. *Trials, Tribulations and Celebration: African-American Perspectives on Health, Illness, Aging and Loss.* Yarmouth, ME: Intercultural Press; 1992:165–170

90. Jamieson RW. Material culture and social death: African-American burial practices. *Hist Archaeol.* 1995;29:39–58

2
Perinatal Health Care Issues
of Old Order Amish Women

Jane S. Wenger

The Amish are a culturally homogeneous population that has maintained strong cultural integrity for more than 3 centuries. They have been characterized as a "high-context" culture in which the members are integrally involved with one another on a personal and community level.[1–3]

Amish society emerged out of the Protestant Reformation in 16th century Europe. As an offshoot of the larger Anabaptist (rebaptizers) movement, which was originated by the Swiss Brethren in Zurich, Switzerland, the Amish became a "separate people" in 1693 under the leadership of Swiss born Jacob Ammann. Through Ammann's preaching of an "uncompromising gospel"[1] and strict adherence to the discipline of the *Meidung* (shunning of the excommunicated) and the *Ordnung* (code of church discipline), Ammann's followers maintained a distinct identity and unity that still exists today. This cultural subgroup is known as the Old Order Amish.[1]

In the 18th and 19th centuries, the Amish emigrated from Europe to America to escape the severe persecution and martyrdom that they suffered as a result of their commitment to pacifism and their failure to acknowledge the state church.[4] Original settlements were made in Pennsylvania; today they have settled throughout North America, with the largest concentrations in rural counties of Pennsylvania, Ohio, Indiana, Iowa, Missouri, and Texas. Other communities exist in several other states and Canada.

Settlements are divided into church districts consisting of approximately 25 to 35 families with a district head, or bishop. "The district is the social and ceremonial unit around which the Amish world orbits... a dense ethnic network."[2] The bishops in a settlement, in turn, form a network that connects the individual districts.

The characteristic appearance of the Old Order Amish is that of the peasants or rural folk in Europe.[1] The clothing styles are dictated by the *Ordnung* and remain unchanged. Amish dress symbolizes humility, modesty, and separateness from the world. Education is limited to the eighth grade because involvement in higher education is considered "worldly" and can lead an individual away from the Amish life.[1] They believe in *Gelassenheit*, or an acceptance of God's will.

Deitsch, or Pennsylvania German, is used in the home and within the Amish community. *Deitsch* is primarily a spoken language and again separates the Old Order Amish from the world.[4]

The Amish reject worldly conveniences such as the ownership of automobiles, engine-powered tractors, telephones, and electricity. The rejection of technology is a means of maintaining separateness and self-sufficiency; they are talented and successful farmers by tradition. Approximately one half of the Pennsylvania Amish are engaged in farming; other trades include carpentry, cabinet making, carriage making, blacksmithing, harness making, and working with lumber. Health/natural food merchandising and the distribution of brand-name herbs and food supplements also can be seen in Amish society, as well as teaching within the Amish school system.[1]

The Amish culture and worldviews are characterized by a strong sense of community. Emphasis is placed on "kinship ties, intergenerational relationships, shared language styles, and deeply held religious values."[5] They attend Sunday services, and silent prayer is observed before meals. Amish settlements are subdivided into church districts, each with 30 to 50 families.[4]

Health and Illness

The Amish are active participants in prevention as well as in acute/chronic illness health care and are committed "to do all one can to help oneself"[4] through the advice of friends and family, alternative and conventional medicine, and folk remedies. Health includes mind, body, and spirit and involves a good appetite, a healthy physical appearance, and a good day's work.[1] "Health and happiness is found in harmony between God, man, and nature."[6] The Amish health care system includes a folk healing art called *brauche*.[4] It is sometimes referred to as "sympathy curing" or "warm hands" and embodies the ability to feel another's pain and suffering. Because there are no professionally trained health care practitioners within the Amish community, "outsiders" must be sought for conventional medical treatment.

An ethnographic study of the phenomenon of caring in an Indiana Amish community identified the behaviors of care that are valued within the Amish culture.[3] Positive values attributed to nurses included "personalized care, visiting, listening, health care instructions, and sensing what is needed." Knowing the culture and demonstrating friendliness, courtesy, and professional competency were also cited as important. Similarly, a caring physician was identified as one who takes time and listens, can be trusted, is competent and moral, is knowledgeable about different treatments and provides information, cares about what the patient thinks, is flexible with payment schedules, and "doesn't ask first about money." The latter 2 traits are particularly important because the Amish generally do not subscribe to health care insurance, and payment for health care services is an individual and/or community responsibility.

The Amish do not readily express their true feelings with strangers; thus the health care provider should try to be nonjudgmental and attempt to elicit their opinions and feelings regarding management options. At times it may seem that they are unwilling to agree to a therapeutic plan or may be unhappy about undertaking the cost of diagnosis and treatment. However, one must take into consideration the effect on the Amish of having to make health decisions in the "worldly" environment. In light of the limited mutual financial aid they give to one another, it is understandable that critical questions would be asked to satisfy the Amish ethic that decisions are made for the good of the community. Honest, sensitive discussion and explanation will usually result in the family's cooperation. Infrequently, a family may wish to discuss the clinical situation and plans of care with their bishop and congregation before making a decision.

Another ethnographic study[7] revealed some commonalties in the utilization of health care by the Amish. Data analysis identified 3 subgroups of health care utilization: those who primarily use conventional health care modalities, those who primarily use alternative health care modalities, and those who use a mixture of conventional and alternative health care modalities. Providers who are familiar with the Amish culture and who will deliver care in the home setting are often sought when conventional medicine is utilized. When this is not possible or when informants were dissatisfied with a particular provider, switches were made in the provider, health care establishment, or in the particular health care modality utilized until suitable care was found. This behavior was consistent across all of the subgroups, as was the use of chiropractic manipulation in varying degrees. Perceptions of conventional medicine as being "strong" medicine was a common theme across the culture, as revealed by Wenger's study.[7] "Strong" medicine seemed to be an expression of both efficacy and safety. The perceived negative effects of conventional medicine were strongest in the alternative modality subgroup and were primarily safety issues based on personal experience with adverse drug reactions and anecdotal reports of negative outcomes associated with conventional drugs.

As a monogamous community, human immunodeficiency virus (HIV), acquired immunodeficiency syndrome (AIDS), and sexually transmitted diseases (STDs) are virtually nonexistent within the Amish community. Their beliefs concerning the birthing process and the care of infants and children have challenged the "state" on several occasions. In 1988 an Amish father was arrested and imprisoned for refusing to continue chemotherapy treatments for his 6-year-old son who had been diagnosed with cancer. The father was uncompromising in his refusal of the treatment because the attending physician had "cursed" God in his presence when he questioned the doctor about the side effects of the chemotherapy. A successful negotiation with the state was made, however, and the father was allowed to choose his son's physician, one who had worked within an Amish community and had knowledge of Amish culture.[8]

Although inbreeding is prevalent within the Amish community, it does not necessarily result in hereditary defects.[1] However, several recessive diseases are common and may account for some deaths in infants; these include dwarfism and associated congenital heart disease, hemophilia B, and phenylketonuria.[4,9]

Pregnancy/Prenatal Care

Large families are prevalent and desired by the Old Order Amish culture. Nevertheless, pregnancy is not openly discussed, and Amish women make an effort to keep others, including their own children, from knowing of an impending birth until physical changes make it obvious.[3,4] Husbands and wives do participate in prenatal classes, but often choose not to participate in sessions when videos are presented.[4]

Although priorities in care were ascribed to pregnant women, infants, and children in all subgroups of the Wenger study,[7] preventive care in the form of prenatal/postnatal care, well-child checkups, and immunizations were sought in varying degrees. Hospital deliveries by physicians were seen more often in the conventional modality utilization subgroup, whereas home births attended by midwives were more common to the alternative modality subgroup.

Labor and Delivery

It is important for the health care provider to realize that Amish women may use herbal preparations to stimulate labor. The laboring woman seldom expresses any discomfort audibly; similarly, while men may be present for birth, they are not likely to be demonstrative, physically or emotionally.[4]

Based on the belief that "childbirth should occur in the home setting in the natural way which God intended,"[8] many Amish women choose to give birth at home or in a homelike setting of a birthing center. Amish communities may recruit lay practitioners and midwives to provide these services. Other Amish women, however, prefer the hospital setting. Rapport with the health care provider and mutual respect for cultural norms are essential in all health care environments.

Postpartum and Newborn Care

After birth, the Amish family prefers to be discharged as soon as possible. This is due to their belief that childbirth is a natural phenomenon and because they probably do not carry health insurance.[4] The postpartum woman receives much assistance from members of the community. The maternal grandmother often comes to stay with the new parents after the birth of their first child. When the new baby is taken to church services for the first time, he or she is welcomed by the congregation and passed from woman to woman.[4]

Family Planning

Children are welcomed into Amish families and viewed as gifts from God; birth control is viewed as interfering with God's will.[1] Despite their reticence to use contraceptives, fertility control is evident among Amish couples. Sterilization, abstinence, withdrawal, and rhythm may be the birth control methods of choice; abortion is not really an option.

Death/Burial Rites

The Amish prefer to die at home surrounded by their close circle of family and friends.[1,4] While death brings an abundance of visitors into the home of the bereaved, the church community takes care of those from a distance and makes all of the funeral arrangements; the burial rites are as simple as all other aspects of Amish life.[4]

Perinatal Health Care Issues of Old Order Amish Women: Key Highlights

Psychosocial/Spiritual Characteristics

- The Amish refrain from public displays of affection.
- They tend to make direct eye contact with others.
- Personal space is respected.
- Women are usually addressed by their first name.
- A handshake greeting is acceptable.
- Although a patient may not agree with the provider, facial expressions will not indicate this.
- They vote "with their feet and their pocketbooks"; while they will not return for health care if displeased, financial considerations shape ultimate decision making.
- Their sense of autonomy is strong, and they are resistant to change.
- Provider choice is influenced by the experience of other Amish friends and family who have been in similar situations.
- The husband and wife will discuss health options; the husband will make the ultimate decision.
- The husband or another female must be in the room if a provider is male.
- Trust is the key element of all provider/client relationships; clients will set the parameters of the relationship on their own terms/timeline.
- Handholding is appropriate as a supportive measure when needed; it should be avoided by a male provider if the husband is not present.
- Teasing is not appropriate; respect for the culture is important.
- Female providers should not touch an adult Amish male; a female provider is preferred for "female issues."

- Amish believe that salvation is dependent on faith, repentance, and baptism.
- Sunday services and prayer are important observances.

Prenatal Care

- There is an increased risk for fetal/child loss because of high fertility rates and increased birth rates with advanced maternal age.
- A woman may present for care at any time during a pregnancy, but usually between the 11th and 12th week for the first pregnancy; it may be later with subsequent pregnancies.
- Preventive care is a foreign concept. Amish women are not opposed to early care, but they do not feel a need for frequent care if they feel well.

Prenatal Testing

- To increase compliance, the rationale for each test or ultrasound should be explained.
- Cost is a major consideration.
- They tend to be resistant to alfa-fetoprotein (AFP) testing.
- Although they are at low risk for HIV, AIDS, and STDs, they will accept prenatal screening as long as it is carried out with sensitivity and discretion.

Pregnancy Diet

- The Amish diet is generally high in sugar and carbohydrates; thus the pregnant woman needs to be reminded about protein intake, especially in the spring when the produce has been harvested. A "lettuce sandwich" is a common meal.
- Processed meats such as bologna, eggs, and cheese are common protein sources.
- They may not drink milk if a particular district does not have refrigeration.
- "Natural" and herbal supplements/teas are popular. The Amish usually take prenatal vitamins during pregnancy.
- Blackstrap molasses is a good source of iron.

Pregnancy-Related Beliefs/Taboos
- Pregnancy and childbirth are not discussed around children; the arrival of a sibling is often a "surprise."
- "Natural" remedies are viewed as safe and are the preferred mode of treatment.
- Herbal products used during pregnancy include red raspberry and chamomile tea, white oak, butcher's broom, sage, goldenseal, acidophilus, and penny royal (which is contraindicated).
- They may use cleansing colonic enemas.
- Conventional medicine is viewed as "strong."
- Immunization from a disease is better than vaccination; this idea is often promulgated by chiropractors.
- They do not like antibiotics, believing they disturb the body's immune system.
- Many believe that reaching over one's head or crawling under a fence can cause the umbilical cord to wrap around the fetus's neck.

Labor and Delivery
- The husband, mother, and/or mother-in-law may be present for the birth. A time for total privacy between husband and wife is needed after the birth.
- Narcotics for pain control and anti-hemorrhagic medications are usually accepted.
- Herbal remedies such as blue/black cohosh, evening primrose, cotton root, and red raspberry tea may be used to enhance uterine contractions.
- Positioning choices vary; generally, the woman ambulates or works during labor.
- A warm shower/whirlpool (if available) is welcomed for relaxation/ discomfort relief.
- The first birth may be in a hospital; a birthing center or home is common for subsequent deliveries, although some still prefer the hospital.

- Some revert to birthing center from home birth when there are older children in the home (privacy issues).
- The laboring woman tends to be provider-dependent; she follows the advice of those she trusts, has past experience with, and who pose no financial concerns.

Postpartum Care
- An "Amish nurse" may be hired for 10 days.
- Some Amish subscribe to 10 days in bed after delivery so that the body organs can "go back in place" by day 9.

Postpartum Diet
- In addition to following the same diet as prenatally, Comfrey tea is thought to help fight infection.

Neonatal Care
- The newborn sleeps in the parents' room until weaned to his or her own crib at night.
- The mother is the caretaker; other female family members help.
- Fussy babies may be taken to the chiropractor or herbalist.
- All newborn boys are circumcised.
- The baby is named after a close Amish friend or family member; the middle name is the mother's maiden name.

Breastfeeding/Breast Care
- New mothers usually breastfeed.

Family Planning
- The contraceptive methods of choice are breastfeeding, withdrawal/ rhythm, natural family planning, foam/condoms, and tubal ligation.
- Most Amish are responsive to the provider's recommendation if contraception will benefit the mother's health and/or increase the chances of a healthy pregnancy post-miscarriage.

Family Involvement
- The woman's mother, mother-in-law, or other female family members help out with the care of the new mother, household, and other children.

Pregnancy Termination/Miscarriage
- The Amish believe that miscarriage, fetal demise, and infant death are God's will.
- They do not blame providers for bad outcomes of pregnancy.
- Abortion is not an option to Amish women.

Death/Burial Rites
- A pregnancy loss is deeply felt because each child is viewed as a gift from God.
- Grieving is private.
- An undertaker's services are used for preparation of the body; viewing is in the home.
- Clocks are stopped at the time of the death.
- Silver dollars are placed over the eyes of the deceased infant.
- Infants are not baptized.
- Infants are not embalmed and are buried within 24 hours of death.
- The Amish usually are not agreeable or receptive to autopsy unless absolutely necessary.

References

1. Hostetler J. *Amish Society*. 4th ed. Baltimore, MD: John Hopkins University Press; 1993
2. Kraybill DB. *The Riddle of Amish Culture*. Baltimore, MD: John Hopkins University Press; 1989
3. Wenger AFZ. *The Phenomenon of Care in a High Context Culture: The Old Order Amish* [dissertation]. Detroit, MI: Wayne State University; 1988/1989
4. Wenger AFZ, Wenger MR. The Amish. In: Purnell LD, Paulanka BJ, eds. *Transcultural Health Care: A Culturally Competent Approach*. Philadelphia, PA: FA Davis; 1998:75–105
5. Wenger AFZ. Cultural context, health and care decision-making. *J Transcultural Nurs*. 1995;7:3–14
6. McGrath WR. *Amish Folk Remedies for Plain and Fancy Ailments*. Rev ed. Cave Creek, CA: Schupp S; 1988
7. Wenger JS. *The Old Order Amish in Pennsylvania: An Ethnographic Study of the Utilization of Alternative Health Care Modalities* [master's thesis]. University Park, PA: Pennsylvania State University, State College; 1999
8. Huntington GE. Health care. In: Kraybill DB, ed. *The Amish and the State*. Baltimore, MD: John Hopkins University Press; 1993:163–189
9. Acheson S. Prenatal, infant, and child death rates among the Old Order Amish. *Am J Epidemiol*. 1994;139:173–183

Acknowledgments

Robert L. Bower, MD, retired family practitioner, Palmyra, PA

Rita Rhodes Martinez, CRNP, CRNM, Birth Care and Family Services, Quarryville, PA

Donna L. Robinson, CRNP, Holms Mortin Clinic for Special Children

Lucille Sykes, Stoneboro, PA

3
Perinatal Health Care Issues of Cambodian Women

Carole Ann Moleti

According to the latest census data,[1] approximately 281.5 million Cambodians live in the United States. They are part of a rapidly growing Asian population that began in the 1970s and now comprises one fourth of the US foreign-born population. Close to one half of Asian immigrants live in major metropolitan areas, with Los Angeles, New York, and San Francisco having the largest representation.[2]

Southeast Asian refugees living in the United States hover at both ends of the socioeconomic spectrum. While 39% of all Asians work in managerial/professional jobs, 53% have health insurance, many have good incomes, and roughly 1 in 8 lives in poverty. In 1990 it was estimated that 1 in 5 year-round, full-time workers earned less than $15,000[3]; 1 decade later, 13% were classified as poor and 17% participated in means-tested assistance programs.[2]

A 1991 US census report indicated that only 37.5% of immigrants from Cambodia were high school graduates, and even those who completed higher education still faced language and cultural barriers[4]; in addition, a significant number were functionally illiterate. More than one third reported that they spoke their native language at home and did not speak English "very well."[4] Reportedly, 51% of Cambodians are married and 23% have children younger than 18 years. The median age of Cambodians in the United States is 35 years[1]; among the women, 39% are aged 18 years or older and 12% live with no spouse, while 7% live with neither spouse nor dependent children.[1] Clearly, this population is in need of perinatal health care services.

The challenges of providing culturally competent health care to foreign-born women and their families lies in understanding, accepting, and respecting their cultural belief systems, customs, experiences and diversities.[5] To develop this competence, the provider must understand the issues that face each immigrant group and learn to work in a way that incorporates the customs and beliefs into the care. This shows respect for the individual and the culture, and facilitates compliance with care.

Most Cambodians are Buddhists. As an outgrowth of the Buddhist religion, there is a belief that human suffering is a part of life.[6,7] Therevada Buddhism emphasizes that the physical body is in unity with the social self and the soul.[8] There is a body-mind-spirit unity, and each part is inseparable from the other.[9] Another health belief is that illness is a form of punishment from angry spirits. To prevent illness, one must live in harmony with the spirits and be mindful of maintaining respect for the balance of all 3.[10] Care that focuses on just physical issues and does not consider or respect the balance will not be meaningful and may not be accepted.[11] It is also important to note that culturally emphasis is placed on stoicism and restraints on public displays of emotions. Women in particular are taught to be quiet and respectful and are often too polite to disagree with health care workers or even abusive or unsupportive partners.[6]

Census data indicate that most Asian families have 5 or more members.[12] In Cambodia, female children are preferred because they can help with household duties, caring for children, and caring for aging parents. However, the strong kinship and support systems that existed in Cambodia often break down following repatriation to the United States. As the younger generations become acculturated to Western culture, they may find themselves in conflict with their more traditional parents. For example, in Cambodia, many marriages are arranged; but young couples may resist this if they have been born and raised in the United States.[13]

Many Cambodian refugees and their children were victims of, or witnesses to, the atrocities of Pol Pot during the 1970s. Some had members of their immediate families openly killed while others had loved ones who just disappeared; many lost their homes and lifestyle when they fled the terrorist regime. As they struggle to rebuild their lives in the United States, they may be afflicted with psychological scars and haunting memories; thus refugees may continue to exhibit sadness over their losses long after they are safe in their new land. Depression, high levels of stress, a lack of social support, and fear of procedures and hospitals have been identified as problems for Cambodian women; in fact, post-traumatic stress disorder (PTSD) is a major mental health issue and may impair social functioning.[13] For women, the events that may have given rise to PTSD include rape and the loss of children, partners, and other family members through death and separation. Despite this, most Cambodians do not seek mental health counseling.[14]

Health and Illness

Culturally and philosophically, Cambodians may have difficulty accepting the Western medical health care system and its biomedical model. Their theories about hot and cold often influence the way they perceive the nature of the illness as well as their judgment toward the treatment prescribed.[6] Health care and hospital access in Cambodia are limited. Whenever possible, Cambodian women prefer female health care providers.

Because polygamy is an accepted practice in Cambodia, it is not uncommon for the men to have several sexual partners. In addition, the hepatitis B virus (HBV) tends to be endemic within the Cambodian community. One study of Southeast Asian refugee teenagers found 14% to be positive for HBV surface antigen and 8% to be chronic carriers.[15] Tuberculosis (TB) is another problem; indeed, the age-specific incidence of bacteriologically confirmed TB in Southeast Asian refugees was found to be much higher than for the US population as a whole.[16] Furthermore, many may be infected with drug-resistant organisms. Hemoglobinopathies are also common within Asian populations. In particular, the carrier frequency for alpha and beta thalassemia and hemoglobin E is quite high, approximating 26%.[17] Thus screening Cambodian immigrants for sexually transmitted diseases (STDs), human immunodeficiency virus (HIV), acquired immunodeficiency syndrome (AIDS), HBV, TB, and blood dyscrasias and therapeutic intervention for those infected are important public health objectives.

Pregnancy/Prenatal Care

In Cambodia there is little, if any, prenatal care, particularly for poor and rural women. Once in the United States, Cambodian women are generally compliant with prenatal care visits, but will be more comfortable with a female provider. However, they are less likely to seek preventive services such as Pap smears, mammography, or smoking cessation programs. They are generally amenable to routine blood testing and sonography, but not amniocentesis.

All pregnant Cambodian women and their family members should be screened for TB, instituting follow-up and treatment of all positive results in accordance with established guidelines. This remains a challenge for perinatal health care providers; however, a culturally acceptable way should be found to ensure compliance. The role of indigenous health care workers who speak *Khmer* has proven to be successful in some settings. If no trained workers are available, other Cambodian patients who have a good command of English should be recruited to assist in the ongoing care and education of those who test positive for TB.

Because there is a high risk for fetuses of thalassemia carriers to develop hydrops fetalis and subsequent blood transfusion–dependent homozygous beta thalassemia, screening Cambodian pregnant women for this hemoglobinopathy is warranted[17]; however, genetic testing will probably be rejected by them and their partners.

There are many dietary practices that affect the health of the pregnant woman and her unborn baby. For example, certain foods are avoided during pregnancy; thus dairy products, which tend to be cold, are not a usual part of the diet. Iron and vitamin pills are also frowned on because they are thought to make the baby too big (V. Nou, personal communication, May 1997). Nutrition education for Cambodian women must, therefore, take into account their general dislike of cheese and dairy products, their propensity toward lactase deficiency, and their preference for highly salted and preserved foods (B. Pederson, personal communication, May 1997).

Superstitions surrounding a woman's activity during pregnancy are also common and may include the following: sesame oil will help to provide for an easier (ie, more slippery) birth, standing in front of a door could cause the baby to get stuck, and bathing during the day can make the baby grow too big (V. Nou, personal communication, May 1997). Sexual activity is generally avoided during the last 3 months of pregnancy because of fears that it will harm the baby (V. Nou, personal communication, May 1997). Because most of their pregnancy-related taboos and beliefs are harmless, health care providers should concentrate on helping the women to appropriately modify harmful behaviors, while respecting their cultural beliefs and practices. Having another Cambodian woman help with the education process may be helpful.

Labor and Delivery

In Cambodia, birth is generally the domain of women, and the men are not involved. Most rural and poorer women deliver at home with traditional birth attendants or village midwives, who learn their trade through apprenticeships (B. Pederson, personal communication, May 1997), making cesarean sections and anesthesia rare. In the larger cities, deliveries occur in the hospitals for those who have money, and the care is usually provided by French-trained physicians (B. Pederson, personal communication, May 1997).

In the United States, couples generally do not attend childbirth classes. While the fathers frequently attend the births, their role is generally more of an observational one. Women prefer to stay at home as long as possible and like to walk around. Cambodian women are always expected to be quiet and dignified. The showing of emotion and loud behavior are seen as serious transgressions.[6] As a result, they tend to be very stoic in labor; quiet moaning tends to be the extent of their manifestation of discomfort. The women are not likely to request analgesia or anesthesia, but they will consider any intervention that is suggested if they trust their birth attendant.

Health care providers should carefully screen all Cambodian women for HBV. Invasive procedures such as fetal scalp electrodes and fetal blood sampling during labor should be avoided in those who test positive.

Postpartum and Newborn Care

Sexual activity during the first 3 months postpartum is prohibited (V. Nou, personal communication, May 1997) and new mothers are not expected to go out or resume most normal activities during this period. In Cambodia, family and friends provide extensive support to women after birth. There is no proscription on bathing. Foods must be hot and spicy. Spices such as garlic, hot pepper, and ginger are believed to help the blood circulate better. Hot poultices made of hot pepper and salt may be applied to the perineum to help healing.

After birth a woman in Cambodia may spend several days resting over a bed of coals where she "roasts" to revive her strength and muscle tone (B. Pederson, personal communication, May 1997). In the United States, rest in bed seems to be an acceptable way to keep warm; however, when an extended family is not available to assist with the other child care and home obligations, it may not be possible for the woman to be afforded this luxury.

Health care providers should be familiar with the current immunization protocols recommended by both the Advisory Committee on Immunization Practices (ACIP) of the Centers for Disease Control and Prevention and the American Academy of Pediatrics and should counsel families accordingly.[15,17,18–20] In 1991 ACIP recommended that "hepatitis B vaccine be integrated into infant vaccination schedules" and that "all unvaccinated children aged <11 years who reside in households of first-generation immigrants where HBV is of high or intermediate endemicity" be vaccinated.[16] Not only should every new mother who has emigrated from Cambodia be encouraged to complete the vaccination series for her infant, but she should be advised that any other exposed family members who are uninfected should also be vaccinated.[15]

Newborn care in Cambodia does not involve any formal religious rites. Circumcision is not done. There is no special prescribed cord care, although a poultice of calcium and goya leaves is sometimes used to protect and cover the fontanels; tiger balm may be used by Cambodian mothers in the United States. Combing the infant's hair is thought to be dangerous to the fontanels and is not done. Routine bathing of the baby is performed. In Cambodia, formula is not readily available and is expensive; thus most women breastfeed. In the United States, however, breastfeeding tends to be shunned by Cambodian immigrants, because formula is readily available and thought to be a status symbol (V. Nou, personal communication, May 1997).

Family Planning

Abortion is not an acceptable option for most Cambodians, even if pregnancy complications are discovered. This is an outgrowth of the Buddhist religion, which views events and incidents as part of the individual's karma (destined path). To artificially interfere in one's karma may result in punishment in a later life. The first duty of the individual is to unerringly fulfill a given role without resistance.[7]

Cambodians tend to have large families. Contraception involving male cooperation (condoms and barrier methods) is usually not accepted. Cambodian women tend to choose methods such as intrauterine devices (IUDs) and contraceptive implants or injectibles that are viewed as easy; oral contraceptives are not feared, but may be seen as too much trouble. Although not routinely performed in Cambodia, surgical sterilizations may be considered by some after emigrating to the United States.

Bioethical Dilemmas

It can be challenging to care for women whose cultural and religious beliefs are different. It is important to remember that many Cambodians have endured an array of physical and psychological hardships, particularly those who were witnesses to violence and/or were in refugee camps. Their approach to health care, pregnancy, and childbirth, in combination with their view of life in general, can be affected by deeply held beliefs as well as traumatic experiences that may overshadow the importance that health care providers place on health care.

Poverty, disease, and high rates of infant and maternal mortality in Cambodia may create a sense of resignation and helplessness among patients. These may be exacerbated in light of their past experiences and traumas. Refugees who come from a background of hardship and deprivation often become accustomed to making do with less than optimal circumstances and may not feel that it is a problem for them. In addition, cultural beliefs about health and disease may make it difficult to convince Cambodians of the importance of certain health interventions, particularly when no physical symptoms of disease are present. For example, ensuring compliance with TB prophylaxis for 6 to 9 months is often difficult if the patient feels well and does not value Western medicines. Similarly, hepatitis B is often asymptomatic, and ensuring vaccination of uninfected family members may require multiple visits. The importance of following these regimens must also be stressed. In cases where communicable diseases may affect others, compliance with care and treatment is critical. Using indigenous staff that speak *Khmer* and can translate the woman's concerns to the provider is essential in situations such as this.

In cases where noncompliance with treatment affects only the individual, the provider has a responsibility to be sure that the patient fully understands the consequences of not performing diagnostic testing. If the patient still does not want to have the testing done, then her choice should be respected and care should be taken to ensure that the patient does not feel that she has shown disrespect to the provider by refusing. This would be a serious behavioral transgression in the Cambodian culture and may result in the patient not returning for further care to avoid confrontation. In all cases where the woman seems reluctant to comply with recommendations, it is helpful to consider what religious, cultural, or non-Western belief systems may be operating. Again, indigenous health care workers can be of great help in areas such as dietary modifications and other treatment options by helping to bridge the gap between the 2 cultures and facilitating a mutually agreeable solution. In so doing, the provider demonstrates that he or she is respectful of the patient's life experiences and beliefs and desires to enhance the trust in the relationship.

Death/Burial Rites

Pregnancy losses at all stages are generally seen as karma. Buddhists believe that all are reborn to new lives. When a child dies, it may be reborn to another family member or given back to its original mother. Stories abound about reincarnation among Cambodian women. It has been told that to identify one child in its future life, one mother removed the toes on one foot before burial. When another child was born missing the identical toes, she believed that her child had been returned. In another instance, a birthmark on a child's leg was noted at death. When another child was born to the same mother with the identical birthmark, it was considered to have been the return of the deceased child. Admiring a baby is also forbidden; if nice things are said, it is believed that evil spirits may come to take the child (V. Nou, personal communication, May 1997).

Every Cambodian Woman Is Unique

Provision of health care to Cambodian women is generally easy and rewarding. It is quite impressive to note the reasonably stable mental health of women who have witnessed such atrocities in their native land. It should be kept in mind that the women may be too polite to disagree or decline services; thus noncompliance is generally one way of dealing with those services that are not desired or deemed to be necessary.

Perhaps it is their religious faith or perhaps it is their community support, but for whatever reason, these women demonstrate resiliency. However, they are often passive and too polite to disagree with health care providers or even partners who are abusive or unsupportive. Thus indigenous health care workers who have a good grasp of the language and culture or other patients who are willing and able to help with translation and interpretation of cultural issues can be helpful resources. Failure to understand and interpret culturally relevant issues can result in provider frustration and decreased access to care for Cambodian women.

Perinatal Health Care Issues of Cambodian Women: Key Highlights

Demographic/Psychosocial/Spiritual Characteristics

- Approximately 281.5 million Cambodians live in the United States.
- The median age of Cambodians in the United States is 35 years.
- Most Cambodians are Buddhists and believe that human suffering is a part of life.
- The Buddhist religion sees events as part of an individual's karma or destined path; to interfere in one's karma may result in punishment in a later life.
- Female children are preferred.
- Women tend to be very polite and nonconfrontational.
- Refugees may exhibit sadness and psychological scars due to memories of terrorism.

- Kinship structure and support systems may be broken down in the United States.
- A significant number of refugees are functionally illiterate.
- Stoicism and emotional restraint are common traits.
- Disease and treatment are often viewed in terms of hot and cold.
- Many parents arrange marriages for their daughters.
- No formal religious ceremony is performed for newborns.

Prenatal Care
- In Cambodia, women receive little if any prenatal care; in the United States, they tend to be compliant.
- Women are unlikely to participate in health screening/counseling programs.
- Indigenous health care workers who speak Khmer can facilitate health care services.
- Female providers are preferred.

Prenatal Testing
- In the United States, sonography and routine blood testing are accepted.
- Screening for STDs, HIV, and AIDS is important; however, HIV screening may not be accepted.
- There is a high carrier frequency of both alpha and beta thalassemia and hemoglobin E.
- Women and partners will usually not consent to genetic counseling/testing or amniocentesis.
- There is a high incidence of HBV; screening of mother and family is important. Fetal scalp sampling and electrodes should be avoided to decrease transmission exposures.
- Drug-resistant TB screening and treatment are important.

Pregnancy Diet
- Cold dairy products are avoided.
- Lactase deficiency is common.
- Highly salted and preserved foods are preferred.

Pregnancy-Related Beliefs/Taboos
- Iron and vitamin pills are thought to make the baby too big.
- Sexual activity is avoided during the last 3 months of pregnancy.
- Standing in front of a door may cause the baby to get stuck.
- Bathing during the day can make the baby grow too big.
- Being cold will make the baby grow too big.
- Sesame oil is commonly used to provide for an easier (slippery) birth.

Labor and Delivery
- Natural childbirth is preferred.
- Women are stoic during birth.
- Women tend to be quiet and dignified.
- Loud behavior is seen as a transgression.
- Positioning is up to the mother and midwife.
- In Cambodia, most women deliver at home.

Postpartum Care
- Routine bathing is resumed and keeping warm is important.
- Women are not expected to work for 3 months.
- Bed rest is thought to be important, but may not be possible without the availability of extended family to help.
- Sexual activity is avoided during the first 3 months postpartum.

Postpartum Diet
- Hot and spicy foods (garlic, hot pepper, and ginger) are believed to help the blood circulate better.

Neonatal Care
- In Cambodia, a poultice of calcium and goya leaves may be used to protect and cover a baby's fontanels; in the United States, tiger balm may be used.
- Combing the baby's hair is avoided because of fear of injuring the fontanels.

- Circumcision is not performed.
- Vaccination against HBV is generally recommended by 2 months of age.

Breastfeeding/Breast Care
- Breastfeeding is the norm in Cambodia.
- In the United States, Cambodians prefer to bottle feed because formula is readily available and thought to be a status symbol.

Family Planning
- IUDs and contraceptive injectibles or implants are preferable.
- Pills are viewed as too much trouble, but are not feared.
- Males do not favor condom or barrier methods.
- Few surgical sterilizations are performed in Cambodia, but may be accepted in the United States.
- Large families are preferred.

Family Involvement
- Men are not involved during labor and delivery in Cambodia, but do participate more in the United States.
- Couples usually do not attend childbirth education classes.
- In Cambodia, family and friends provide extensive support so that the women can avoid normal activities for 3 months after the birth; this help may not be available in the United States.

Pregnancy Termination/Miscarriage
- Abortion is not usually considered, even with pregnancy problems.

Bioethical Dilemmas
- Direct refusal of a medical regimen would show disrespect for the implied authority of the provider and is not an acceptable behavior for Cambodian women.
- Noncompliance with recommended care or failure to return for care may indicate a conflict between what the provider recommends versus religious/traditional beliefs or customs.

- Women may choose non-Western treatments, such as herbal preparations, and may decline prescription medications.
- Securing a Cambodian woman's cooperation in treatment and vaccination protocols for infectious diseases such as TB and hepatitis B may require counseling in Khmer by another Cambodian woman to ensure compliance.
- When the recommended care has implications for the patient and the fetus only (genetic concerns), the patient's wishes should be respected while ensuring that she understands the implications of declining genetic counseling/amniocentesis.
- Care should be taken that the woman does not perceive that the provider is impatient or angry at her for not following treatment recommendations.

Death/Burial Rites
- Buddhists believe that all are born to new lives after death.
- Children who die are expected to be returned in another life to the mother or a close family member.
- If nice things are said about the baby, it is believed that evil spirits may take the child away.

References

1. United States Census 2000. *American Fact Finder.* Available at: http://www.USCensus.gov. Accessed February 1, 2003
2. United States Census. *Community Population Survey: Profile of the Foreign Born Population, 2000.* Available at http://www.USCensus.gov. Accessed February 1, 2003
3. US Department of Commerce. *Census Bureau Releases 1990: Census Counts of Specific Racial Groups.* Washington, DC: Bureau of the Census; 1991. CB 91 215
4. US Department of the Census. *Current Population Reports: Population Characteristics in the Asian and Pacific Islander Population in the United States, March 1990 and 1991.* Washington, DC: US Government Printing Office; 1992
5. Rowe JL, Paine L, Barger MK. Primary care for women: cultural competence in primary care services. *J Nurse Midwif.* 1996;41:92–100

6. Lin-Fu J. Asian and Pacific Islander Americans: an overview of demographic characteristics and health care issues. *Asian Am Pacific Islander
   J Health.* 1993;1:20–36
7. Frazier A. *Buddhism: Readings in Eastern Religious Thought.* Philadelphia,
   PA: Westminster Press; 1969
8. Ong A. Making the biopolitical subject: Cambodian immigrants, refugee
   medicine and cultural citizenship in California. *Soc Sci Med.*
   1995;40:1243–1257
9. Thich NH. *Being Peace.* 3rd ed. London, UK: Random House; 1987
10. Buchwald D, Panwala S, Hooten TM. Use of traditional health practices
    by Southeast Asian refugees in a primary care clinic. *West J Med.*
    1992:156:507–511
11. Downs K, Bernstein J, Marchese T. Providing culturally competent
    primary care for immigrant and refugee women: a Cambodian case
    study. *J Nurse Midwif.* 1997;42:499–508
12. United States Census. *Asian and Pacific Islander Population in the United
    States: Current Population Survey, March 2000 Update.* Available at:
    http://www.USCensus.gov. Accessed February 1, 2003
13. Mollica R, Wyshak G, Lavalle J. The psychological impact of war trauma
    torture on Southeast Asian refugees. *Am J Psychiatry.* 1987;144:1567–1572
14. Carlson EB. Mental health status of Cambodian refugees ten years after
    leaving their homes. *Am J Orthopsychiatry.* 1993;63:223–231
15. Centers for Disease Control and Prevention. Hepatitis B virus: a com-
    prehensive strategy for eliminating transmission in the United States
    through universal childhood vaccination—recommendations of the
    Immunization Practices Advisory Committee. *MMWR Morb Mortal
    Wkly Rep.* 1991;40:1–24
16. Farrar LS. Tuberculosis among Indochinese refugees in the United States.
    JAMA. 1983;249:1455–1460
17. Crocker AC, ed. *Thalassemia in Southeast Asian Refugees: Public Health
    Planning Aspects. Report of a Conference at Irvine, CA/Boston MA,
    Children's Hospital.* 1985
18. American Academy of Pediatrics Committee on Infectious Diseases.
    Universal hepatitis B immunization. *Pediatrics.* 1992;89:795–800
19. US Department of Health and Human Services, Public Health Services,
    National Center for Infectious Diseases. Viral hepatitis B recommenda-
    tions. *MMWR Morb Mortal Wkly Rep.* 1995;44:574–575
20. American Academy of Pediatrics Committee on Infectious Diseases.
    Recommended childhood immunization schedule—United States,
    January–December, 2003. *Pediatrics.* 2003;111:212. Available at
    http://www.aap.org/policy/0212.htm. Accessed July 15, 2003

4
Perinatal Health Care Issues of Chinese Women

Yu-Ling Lai and Lily S. Y. Hsia

Asian Americans belong to the fastest-growing ethnic group in the United States. Restrictive laws of the 19th and early 20th centuries excluded Asians from US immigration; however, the 1965 Immigration Act reopened the gates, allowing 20,000 immigrants from each country to enter every year.[1] Since then the growth of the Asian American population has been dramatic. In 1960 there were only 877,934 Asians in the United States, representing a mere 1% of American people; 30 years later, they numbered about 7 million, or 3% of the population.[1] By the year 2000 Asian Americans will probably represent 4% of the total US population. In California, Asian Americans already make up 10% of the state's inhabitants.[1]

In 1850 only 1,000 Chinese inhabited the United States; by 1880, this figure grew to more than 100,000, mostly men, due to the discovery of gold in California and the need for cheap labor to build the transcontinental railroads.[2] In 1990 the Census Bureau reported more than 1.6 million members of the Chinese American community living in the United States.[1] It is further estimated that an additional 400,000 ethnic Chinese reside in the United States today.[1] Most Chinese are first-generation immigrants who came to this country mainly from China, Taiwan, Hong Kong, and Southeast Asian countries during the past 2 decades. A large percentage of this population can be found in the "Chinatowns" of New York City and California.

Chinese culture teaches the concept of family harmony and values obedience; it is believed that arguing and creating conflict brings dishonor to families. Thus many Chinese exhibit a passive and accepting demeanor. Emotions are seldom expressed in public, even when coping with illness and death. The male members of the Chinese family tend to have more power and authority over the females. A variety of religions are observed throughout China; however, Atheism predominates within the People's Republic of China.

Health and Illness

With Chinese Americans making up such a substantial portion of the American population, it is clearly desirable for the modern health care professional to be informed about the relationship between health and culture among the Chinese. Only with this understanding will the needs of this ethnic group be able to be met effectively. For example, studies of eating habits reveal a culturally based lack of dairy intake. The Chinese diet does not include many "traditional" American dairy products such as milk, cheese, or cream. (See Table 4-1.) This exclusion of dairy products dates back to ancient China, as does a long history of lactose intolerance. Many Chinese women who have attempted to integrate dairy products into their diets report the classic symptoms of lactose intolerance; others simply do not like the taste of milk. Alpha thalassemia, a hereditary anemia, is also relatively common among the Chinese[3]; thus careful nutritional and hematologic screening is very important among this population.

A key to understanding Chinese attitudes toward health and nutrition lies in the ancient belief in the Yin and the Yang, the 2 opposing natural forces that must be balanced for peace and harmony. (See Box 4-1.) The Yin, corresponding to cold, darkness, emptiness, and wetness, must be opposed equally by the Yang, corresponding to warmth, brightness, fullness, and dryness.[2] Everything from diet to room temperature must be taken into consideration. Only by carefully balancing the Yin and the Yang, and evenly distributing body heat, say the Chinese, can optimal health be attained. Acupuncture, moxibustion (application of heat), and herbal remedies are among the traditional methods of health restoration commonly employed by the Chinese.[2] (See Table 4-2.)

Table 4-1
Common Food Choices Among Chinese Women*

Protein	Dairy	Grains	Vegetables	Fruits	Fats & Oils	Other
Squid	Cow milk	White rice	Bamboo shoots	Apples	Chicken fat	Seasonings
Fresh, salted, or preserved Fish	Condensed milk	Enriched and non-enriched rice	Bean sprouts	Bananas	Coconut oil	Anise, ginger
Shrimp		Wheat flour	Beets	Cantaloupe‡	Lard	Cilantro, garlic
Oysters		Glutenous rice	Celery	Carambola (star fruit)†	Corn oil	Cooking wine, salt
Abalone		Noodles	Cabbage†	Cherries	Canola oil	Pepper, corn starch
Crab		White bread	Chayote	Dates	Peanut oil	Fermented black beans, vinegar
Scallops		Oatmeal	Napa cabbage†	Grapes	Vegetable oil	Scallions
Pork		Barley	Scallions, onions	Grapefruit†	Sesame oil	Sesame oil, sugar
Chicken		Spaghetti	Coriander	Honeydew		Sauces
Pigeon eggs		Macaroni	Cucumbers	Kumquats		Chili sauce
Beef		Rice noodles	Long green beans	Lime		Soy sauce
Organ meats		Tapioca	Kohlrabi	Loquats		Bean paste
Duck			Leeks	Lychee†		Hoisin sauce
Tofu			Lily blossoms	Oranges†		Sweet & sour sauce
			Bitter melon	Mangoes‡		Oyster sauce
			Mustard greens‡	Papayas‡		Chinese mustard
			Hairy melon	Peaches		Snacks
			Winter melon	Passion fruit		Watermelon seeds
			Snow peas	Pears		
			Chinese turnips	Persimmons§		
			Chinese mushrooms	Pineapples†		
				Plums		

Table 4-1
Common Food Choices Among Chinese Women*, *continued*

Protein	Dairy	Grains	Vegetables	Fruits	Fats & Oils	Other

			Taro
			Tomato†
			Water chestnuts
			Jicama
			Lotus roots
			Ginkgo
				Sugar cane
				Strawberries†
				Tangerines
				Watermelon
						Cookies, candy
						Crackers
						Fresh &
						    preserved
						    fruits, peanuts
						Almonds,
						    cashews
						Tea, soy milk
						Sweet tea

*Source: Cross-Cultural Nutrition Counseling: Massachusetts' Nutrition Assistant (CPA1) Training Guide Commonwealth of Massachusetts, Department of Public Health, WIC Program, March 1997.

†A source of vitamin C >20 mg per serving.

‡A source of Vitamin C >20 mg per serving and Vitamin A >2,500 IU per serving.

§A source of vitamin A >2,500 IU per serving.

Box 4-1
Hot and Cold/Yin and Yang

Foods have special meaning for all ethnic and cultural groups. This is especially true for the Chinese, who have a traditional belief system of "hot" and "cold" foods. This tenet goes along with the Yin and Yang assumption that for an individual with a hot disease, balance must be reached by having cold foods, and vice versa, because disease is seen as a manifestation of disharmony and disruption of the body's equilibrium. In daily life, one needs to balance the interior process of nurturing the self (Yin) with the challenges of the outside world at large (Yang). To overwork, get too much exercise, and excessively engage in activities is to overindulge the Yang, which leads to Yin depletion. The consequences of this may be muscle and joint pains, fatigue, or overexertion on heart and kidneys. However, being overly protective (nourishing the interior of the body by not doing physical exercise or any exertion, which weakens the muscles and stiffens the joints) produces an overabundance of Yin.[4] The theory of Yin and Yang is grounded in traditional Chinese medicine. One of the essential beliefs of the Chinese is that all things in the universe are either Yin or Yang but there are no absolutes—in other words, nothing is ever all Yin or all Yang, but a balance between the 2 forces.

Yin is associated with things that are dark, passive, and cold. Female, night, moist, cold, winter, death, small, and solid are a few examples of Yin. Yang is associated with brightness, warmth, and motion. Male, day, dry, hot, summer, birth, large, and hollow are some examples of Yang. Each organ system has elements of Yin and Yang within it.

The treatment of disease not only uses herb remedies and dietary treatments, but also incorporates therapies such as acupuncture, Tai chi and massage therapy. These are all treatment modalities the Chinese use to correct imbalances in the body.

Diet therapies are based on the belief that specific health problems are caused by dietary imbalance. Traditional Chinese medicine classifies foods into 3 groups: cold/cool foods, neutral foods, and warm/hot foods.

The cold/cool foods have the medicinal functions of clearing heat and fire, cooling the blood, and eliminating toxins. Foods considered cold/cool are watermelon, salad greens, ice cream, bananas, avocados, cold and raw foods, and liquids. Other cold/cool foods include excessive alcohol, animal fats, processed or artificially preserved foods, dairy produce, wheat, yeast, barley, millet, buckwheat, green beans, celery, spinach, green cabbage stems, white turnips, bamboo shoots, lily bulbs, lotus roots, eggplant, tomato, white gourd, sponge gourd, cucumber, bitter melon, apple, pear, orange, rabbit meat, frog meat, duck meat, crab, fresh water snail, kelp, laver, green tea, soy sauce, table salt, and rock candy.

Box 4-1
Hot and Cold/Yin and Yang, *continued*

The warm/hot foods serve to warm the meridians or the energy channels and thus strengthen the Yang, invigorating the blood, opening collateral meridians, and getting rid of the cold. Foods that promote Yang include glutinous rice, Chinese sorghum, pumpkin, hot pepper, ginger, scallions, onions, leeks, funnel greens, garlic, parsley, mustard greens, dates, walnut kernels, plums, peaches, pomegranates, cherries, apricots, chestnuts, pineapples, alcoholic spirits, vinegar, black tea, pepper, coffee, chicken, turkey, mutton, venison, spotted silver carp, grass fish, trout, and red sugar.

Neutral foods are used to act as bridges, harmonizing or neutralizing the diet to bring about a balanced state. Neutral foods in-clude polished rice, wheat, corn, soybeans, peas, small red beans, cauliflower, carrots, wood ears, mushrooms, yams, day lily buds, peanuts, potatoes, lemons, grapes, olives, lotus seed, pork, beef, goose meat, spring chicken, pigeon meat, quail meat, eggs, quail eggs, carp, mandarin fish, eel, yellow croaker, turtle, jelly fish, abalone, white sugar, honey, jasmine tea, and oolong tea.[5]

Newer generations of younger immigrants and first- or second-generation Chinese born in America seem to accept Chinese folk and Western medicine. The longer these newer generations live in this country, the more likely they are able to adapt to Western culture and its health care practices. Chinese immigrants tend to accept caregiver instructions and obey without question, except if a practice is contrary to a firmly held belief system.

Pregnancy/Prenatal Care

Chinese culture views pregnancy as a natural condition beyond human control even if the child is impaired. Because the Chinese tend to believe that aborted (or miscarried) fetuses do not belong to the family, they usually will not show any emotional reaction following an abortion or miscarriage.

In 2000 US census data revealed that 87.6% of Chinese mothers began their prenatal care in the first trimester compared with 83.2% for all races.[1] That same year only 2.2% of Chinese women either

Table 4-2
Herbs Commonly Used by the Chinese[4–8]

Botanical Name	English/Chinese Common Name	Conditions Treated and/or Intended Actions
Zingiber officinale	Ginger	Relieve morning sickness, nausea, and vomiting
Angelica sinensis	Dong Quai (Angelica)	Regulate menstrual rhythm, strengthen the womb including dysmenorrhea, oligomenorrhea, premenstrual and menopausal syndrome
Astragalus membranceus	Huang Qi (Astragalus root)	Support immunocompromised body system undergoing radiation and chemotherapy, common cold/sore throat, fatigue, hepatitis, liver support, increase stamina and endurance
Schisandra chinensis	Wu Wei Zi (Schisandra)	Strengthen uterine contractions, promote dilatation of the cervix, allay fatigue, and alleviate chronic cough and asthma, insomnia, diarrhea, thirst, fatigue, sexual debility, and memory loss
Poria cocos	Fu Ling	Relieve abdominal distention, dyspepsia, edema, difficulty in urination, diabetes and diarrhea
Ginkgo biloba	Ginkgo	Improve memory and learning, increase blood flow especially in the capillaries
Allium sativum	Garlic	Useful in altitude sickness, arthritis, athlete's foot, fighting colds and flu; lowers blood pressure and cholesterol
Panax ginseng	Ginseng	Boost immunity, increase energy and vigor, helpful during convalescence
Camellia sinensis	Green Tea	Relieve stomach disorders, vomiting, and diarrhea

started their prenatal care in the third trimester or received no prenatal care, while the same was true for 3.9% of the total population.[1]

The Chinese culture encourages the use of special food selections for women during pregnancy and after delivery. Nevertheless, calcium deficiency is often seen in women[9]; indeed, studies have shown that, regardless of their educational or socioeconomic background, the Chinese tend to have calcium insufficiency problems before and during pregnancy as well as during the postpartum breastfeeding period. This has adverse effects on calcium and mineral levels in maternal and fetal blood, as reflected in the common expression that for each baby delivered, the baby will "eat up" one of the mother's teeth.

In addition to calcium, Chinese women may also have inadequate intakes of iron, phosphate, and vitamins A, B_2, and niacin.[9] Despite the need for calcium and minerals in fetal development, ensuring adequate calcium intake can be difficult due to the high percentage of Asian people who are lactose intolerant.[10] This is often manifested by diarrhea, gas, and bloating problems following the consumption of even small amounts of dairy products. In such cases, dietary consultation may be necessary. Alternate food supplements, such as soybean products, can provide good choices to them in supplying appropriate nutrition, particularly for protein and calcium. Primigravidas tend to be more conscious of their nutrition balance and food intake than multigravidas.[9] Thus reinforcement of nutrition education becomes very important in the care of Chinese women during subsequent pregnancies.

An important antenatal issue is anemia. In addition to their propensity for alpha thalassemia,[3] most Chinese women do not eat much iron-rich red meat, preferring rice, fish, and vegetables instead. Due to the insufficient amounts of iron present in these foods, iron supplementation may be necessary. However, once they experience side effects such as constipation or diarrhea, they may stop taking the supplements without consulting the health care provider. This response is rooted in the Chinese philosophy that happiness and contentment must be taken into account when assessing everything from family dynamics to health.[11]

Thus if discomfort accompanies administration of a drug or therapy, the Chinese exert their right to stray from "orders" in favor of restoring "normalcy." This contrasts with the attitude that is more prevalent in the Western world that one must strictly adhere to a prescribed regimen, confident that any side effects can be weathered in the pursuit of restored health.

Labor and Delivery

In older generations, Chinese men were not allowed to be present during labor. This was based on the belief that postpartum blood and the placenta were dirty materials and would bring bad luck to a man. However, the newer generations are more inclined to view support from the husband as an essential component to a successful labor. Still, many Chinese women prefer female companions during birth. In general, Chinese couples do not attend childbirth classes.

The old idea that women must eat a good meal to have energy to push during labor may still influence women today. It is worth emphasizing to patients that a full stomach may cause nausea and vomiting toward the end of labor and could be problematic should general anesthesia be required in an emergency.

Postpartum and Newborn Care

Since ancient times, the postpartum period has been granted a very special status in Chinese culture. Although women received no reprieve from their household chores during pregnancy, following birth they expected, and were granted, ample time to recover and return to full strength. Today the state of postpartum health is still believed to be ultimately responsible for a woman's health status in middle age and even old age. The postpartum woman, then, is encouraged to take plenty of time to recover, and is not expected to resume her full workload immediately. Her body is at a delicate turning point; if not treated with the utmost care, she may become highly susceptible to illness. Some examples of "women's diseases" classically linked to poor postpartum care by Chinese physicians include chronic arthritis, backaches, joint pain, incontinence, and vaginal discharge.[12] Although the maternal grandmother is the preferred companion during the postpartum period, parents from both sides may be willing to help during the first month.

In the United States, the Chinese seem to adapt readily to the Western culture of "pampering" women during pregnancy. Indeed, mothers-to-be are often encouraged to stay off their feet, allowing others to take over the heavier housework; they may even take a leave of absence from work well in advance of their due dates. Once the child is born, however, they are usually expected to return home within 2 to 3 days after the birth and become active soon thereafter.

The Chinese do not name their babies after their parents out of respect for their memory. In fact, it is considered disrespectful to name a baby after anyone they love. There is no difference regarding circumcision beliefs between Chinese and Western cultures. Although some people think it is unnecessary, there is no prohibition against circumcising a newborn boy.

The rate of breastfeeding among Chinese women varies. Despite the known benefits of breast milk, many new mothers choose to bottle-feed their babies for convenience sake, particularly because they tend to return to work so soon after giving birth. In addition, some women believe that infant formula is more nutritious.

The traditional adherence to the "laws of nature" may lead to some potentially harmful practices among Chinese women, at least according to the standards of traditional Western postpartum care. The Chinese believe that a woman's pores are open in the postpartum period, leaving her subject to even the slightest draft (called "wind"), or worse, the countless diseases present in a hospital.[12] Thus she may dress too warmly, insist on keeping all doors and windows closed, and avoid fans or air-conditioning. Because birth is believed to result in a huge loss of body heat, catching a cold may be viewed as a serious health threat. As a result, the postpartum Chinese woman may often refuse to leave the warmth of her bed for several days. Some women may stay in bed for a whole month to 45 days following delivery. Because of this belief, women recovering from cesarean section may refuse to get out of bed on the second day.

Chinese women who believe in the Yin and the Yang[12] also strictly regulate bathing. Water, like wind, is always considered "cold," regardless of its actual temperature; thus some postpartum women refuse to bathe lest they lose body heat. Any contact with water, including showering, hand washing, or even dishwashing, is seen as a potential source of cold. Only water that is extremely hot, or infused with a "hot" substance like ginger, is deemed acceptable for use by some.

Also, according to the Yin and the Yang concept, foods that are considered "cold" should not be consumed following pregnancy; instead, only those believed to be "hot" should be eaten. (See Box 4-1.) The essence, rather than the physical temperature of the food, is used to define hot and cold. The desire to avoid "cold" foods often leads to refusal of, or selective eating from, hospital trays.[13] Potentially, this could lead to a poorly balanced diet and vitamin or mineral deficiencies. Constipation is commonly seen in Chinese postpartum women due to the consumption of a diet that may lack vegetables (fiber) and sufficient water. Herbal diets are an important issue in the postpartum period. Women are told to eat certain foods that are prepared by adding a variety of Chinese herbs.

Other postpartum restrictions are commonly followed. For example, women are advised that reading and crying during the postpartum period because they will damage their vision, and that stair climbing and consuming nuts or high-sodium foods can be very harmful to their health.[14]

Family Planning

There are no differences in family planning issues between the Chinese and Western cultures. The use of condoms, intrauterine devices (IUDs), and birth control pills are the most common contraceptive choices by Chinese couples.

Retaining the family's last name is very important to Chinese families; thus the birth of a male infant is highly valued. For this reason, there are many methods used by Chinese couples to attempt to conceive a male infant, including the adherence to special food selections and/or the observance of herbal medicine. Because female infants are traditionally less valued than male infants, care may need to be taken in helping a family value a baby girl. In mainland China, a disproportionate number of female fetuses are aborted.

Bioethical Dilemmas

Health care is a dynamic, interactive process in which each party—the care provider and the patient—brings a set of cultural beliefs, religious and social practices, and expectations to the encounter. Sometimes a common understanding is reached when there is a concern, diagnosis, or intervention that needs to be addressed and followed. Other times, despite the agreement by both parties, differences persist as to what should be done about the problem. When the health care provider and the patient share similar beliefs on health and illnesses, the encounter or the health care visit usually is smooth and satisfying for both. When the basic assumption on what causes the illness is diverse, and there are differences in cultural beliefs on what the expected treatment should be, not only is there a clash of value systems, but the intervention could potentially be ineffective and unsatisfactory to both.

One of the practices that is strongly held and firmly adhered to by women for generations in China is that after giving birth, the postpartum woman is expected to be "sitting for a month" or resting for a whole month at home to restore her health and prevent future illness occurring in old age. It is believed that after delivery, the blood from a woman's womb is unclean and offensive; therefore she must remain at home. It is unacceptable for her to visit or worship in the temples or to see visitors and friends. Usually the woman's mother, her mother-in-law, or a nanny will care for her and her baby during the entire first month postpartum. Often the mother and infant are together only during breastfeeding. Western providers may feel there is little opportunity for mother-infant bonding or that these actions imply that the mother is not interested in her newborn.

Based on the concept of Yin and Yang, the postpartum woman is believed to be in a state of Yin. She should not go out of the house to meet the wind, which would affect her bones and joints in her old age with rheumatism or chronic joint pains. She should not bathe or wash her hair because the vital force within her body is in a state of imbalance at this time. Drinking cold water is to be avoided as are "cold" foods such as Chinese cabbage, green beans, turnips, bamboo shoots, leafy vegetables, and most fruits. The diet is dominated by "hot" foods such as chicken prepared with sesame seed oil and rice wine, pork and pork livers, kidneys, and eggs, which supply excessive protein and fat. These high-fat, and high-protein foods, with few fruits and vegetables, constitute the postpartum woman's daily intake. The cultural beliefs of immigrant Chinese women and many of the taboos they and their families adhere to are often in conflict with Western practices. Health care providers may have problems with Chinese patients regarding cultural traditions of hygiene and dietary habits.

In China most doctors have some training in both Western and Chinese traditional medicine. Most of the hospitals there are accustomed to offering patients the choice of Western medicine or traditional medicine. Less than a hundred years ago, the health care system in China was predominately based on folk medicine. The Chinese believe that the human body is a gift from the ancestors and it should be revered, well cared for, and carefully maintained. When the body's life force and energy are sluggish and out of balance, herbs and special remedies are used to correct specific ailments. Immigrants from China are so accustomed to the traditional herbs as a mode of treatment that many patients will return to China for herbal, acupuncture, or massage treatment if the Western medicine or surgery performed in the United States does not yield satisfactory results to the expectations of the patients.[15]

When a sonogram is done on the pregnant woman for determination of gestational age and evaluation of the fetus for any abnormalities, Chinese women will frequently ask whether the sonogram shows the gender of the unborn child. Many mothers-in-law and husbands would like to have a male child as their firstborn. For centuries, male babies have been highly valued in this patriarchal and traditional society. The gender preference in China with the current "one-child family" national policy puts a heavy burden on the pregnant woman. When a woman is told by the provider that the gender of the baby is not generally evaluated or reported as a part of the sonogram report, the expectant woman not only is disappointed, but she may even go to another doctor just to seek information on whether her baby is a boy or a girl.

Some newly immigrated Chinese families in which husbands and wives are working will send their newborns to the Republic of China (mainland China) to be cared for by the child's grandparents, aunts, or other relatives. The cost of child care and food is lower in China compared with the United States. When children reach school age, they are sent back to their parents in the United States. There are many complex social and family issues facing these children because they have been uprooted from what they know, do not really know their parents, do not speak English, and must adjust to a new country—even if it is the country of their birth.

Death/Burial Rites
In ancient China, children have to be 18 years old to be accepted as adults. If a child dies before he or she reaches adulthood, parents will

not plan any formal ceremonies. Chinese people believe that parents should die before their children. The cultural belief is that letting gray hair (parents) arrange a funeral for black hair (children) will add more sin to this dead person. The Chinese believe that if parents ritualize the death of a child, that child's transmigration to a new life will be plagued by bad fortune. In addition, a fetus or baby that has died should not be considered as a family member. When death occurs in a Chinese family, they tend to minimize any ceremony or recognition of the event, such as pictures, naming the baby, or even funeral arrangements. They do not forget the experience. It is simply seldom discussed in public. When dealing with death, the medical caregiver must be very careful in evaluating the needs of the parents. Too much ritual imposed by the caregiver may cause significant anxiety for the family. Rituals should be presented as an option. A nonjudgmental attitude is more helpful to parents who want to deal with loss in their own way. However, safeguards against suicide may be necessary following infant death. Grief may be much deeper than articulated when added to the sorrows/traumas of an earlier life and the separation/isolation imposed by emigration.

Every Chinese Woman Is Unique

Provision of health care to Chinese women is generally quite easy and rewarding. They are often too polite to disagree with medical interventions; however, health care workers must be sensitive to and accepting of those alternative belief systems and cultural norms that do not pose a danger to the mother or baby. There should always be access to Chinese translators who can also help with the interpretation of cultural issues when appropriate. Failure to understand and interpret culturally relevant issues can result in provider frustration and decreased compliance by Chinese women.

Perinatal Health Care Issues of Chinese Women: Key Highlights

Demographic/Psychosocial/Spiritual Characteristics

- It is estimated that 2 million ethnic Chinese reside in the United States today.
- Most Chinese immigrants are first-generation immigrants who came to this country mainly from China, Taiwan, Hong Kong, and Southeast Asian countries during the past 2 decades.
- A large percentage of Chinese can be found in the "Chinatowns" of New York City and California.
- Family harmony is highly valued.
- Deep respect is held for the male role in the family.
- Obedience to one's elders is strictly observed.
- Emotions are seldom expressed in public.
- The forces of Yin (cold, darkness, emptiness, and wetness) must be balanced with those of Yang (warmth, brightness, fullness, and dryness) in all aspects of life.

Prenatal Care

- Patients tend to accept caregiver instructions and obey without question.
- Pregnancy is viewed as a natural condition beyond human control and should not be tampered with by too much human interference.
- A high percentage of Chinese women begin their prenatal care during the first trimester.

Prenatal Testing

- Amniocentesis and chorionic villus sampling are not likely to be accepted.
- Alpha thalassemia is relatively common among the Chinese population; thus patient screening is very important.

Pregnancy Diet

- Lactose intolerance is common, and dairy products may be avoided; thus dietary counseling on alternative food supplements may be necessary to avoid calcium, phosphate, and vitamins A, B_2, and niacin deficiencies.
- Chinese women may not eat nuts or consume high-sodium foods.
- Iron deficiency anemia is prevalent among pregnant Chinese women; although iron supplements should be considered, side effects such as constipation or diarrhea may interfere with compliance.

Pregnancy-Related Beliefs/Taboos

- Women are warned not to move their households or remodel their homes during pregnancy.
- Pregnant women should not consume coffee, tea, and spices.
- Optimal health in pregnancy can only be attained by carefully balancing the Yin and the Yang and evenly distributing body heat.

Labor and Delivery

- In general, Chinese couples do not attend childbirth classes.
- Women believe that they must eat a good meal to have energy to push during labor.

Postpartum Care

- The quality of postpartum health is believed to be ultimately responsible for a woman's health in middle age and even old age; if she does not take time to recover and rest adequately, she may become highly susceptible to such illnesses as chronic arthritis, backaches, joint pain, incontinence, and vaginal discharge. (See Box 4-1.)
- Chinese women may choose to bathe only in very hot water or water infused with ginger.
- Prolonged postpartum bed rest lasting anywhere from a month to 45 days may be observed.

Postpartum Diet
- Foods that are "cold" should not be consumed following pregnancy; instead, only "hot" foods such as chicken soup, rice, or eggs should be eaten.
- Nuts and foods high in sodium are thought to harm one's health when consumed after birth and generally are avoided.

Neonatal Care
- Chinese do not name their babies after their parents as a means of expressing respect for their memory.
- Although some believe it unnecessary, there is no prohibition in the Chinese culture against circumcising the newborn boy.

Breastfeeding/Breast Care
- The rate of breastfeeding varies among Chinese women; working women often choose formula supplements.
- Some believe that infant formula is more nutritious than breast milk.

Family Planning
- The use of condoms, IUDs, and birth control pills are popular.
- Because a male infant is preferred to keep the family's name, some try different methods to have a male infant (eg, eating particular foods and using herbal medicine).

Family Involvement
- Female companions are preferred during birth; however, the newer generations believe support from the husband is an essential component of a successful labor and delivery.
- The maternal grandmother is the preferred companion during the postpartum period; however, parents from both sides may be willing to help during the first month.

Pregnancy Termination/Miscarriage
- A perfect (normal) pregnancy is highly valued; termination of an abnormal fetus will likely be chosen.
- Families believe that aborted fetuses do not belong to the family; thus the individual family members may not express sadness and emotions of grief, especially in public.

Bioethical Dilemmas
- The cultural beliefs of immigrant Chinese women and many of the taboos they and their families adhere to are often in conflict with Western practices.
- Health care providers may have problems with Chinese patients regarding cultural traditions of hygiene and dietary habits.

Death/Burial Rites
- The Chinese rarely ritualize the death of a child.
- Care should be taken to observe serious "masked" depression in cases of infant loss.

References

1. Martin JA, Hamilton BE, Ventura SJ, Menacker F, Park MM. Births: final data for 2000. *Nat Vital Stat Rep.* 2002;505:55. Available at: http://www.sfusd.k12.ca.us/schwww/sch405/IUP/popDistribut.html. Accessed February 15, 2003
2. Spector RE. *Cultural Diversity in Health and Illness.* 5th ed. Upper Saddle River, NJ: Prentice Hall Health; 2000
3. Matocha LK. Chinese-Americans. In: Purnell LD, Paulanka BJ, eds. *Transcultural Health Care: A Culturally Competent Approach.* Philadelphia, PA: FA Davis; 1998:163–188
4. Beinfield H, Korngold E. *Between Heaven and Earth: A Guide to Chinese Medicine.* New York, NY: Ballantine Books; 1991
5. Medboo Health. *Traditional Chinese Dietotherapy.* 1999. Available at: http://www.ontcm.com/healthy/foods.htm. Accessed February 15, 2003
6. *PDR for Herbal Medicines.* Montvale, NJ: Medical Economics; 1998
7. Chmelik S. *Chinese Herbal Secrets.* Garden City Park, NY: Avery Publishing Group; 1999
8. Duke JA. *Dr. Duke's Essential Herbs.* New York, NY: St Martin's Press; 1999

9. Chang SJ. Studies on the nutrient intake of pregnant and lactating women from Taiwan area. *J Chinese Nutr Soc.* 1991;16:101–118

10. Tadataka Y. *Textbook of Gastroenterology.* Vol 2. Philadelphia, PA: JB Lippincott; 1991:1521–1522

11. Anderson JM. Health across cultures. *Nurs Outlook.* 1990;38:136–139

12. Pillsbury BLK. Doing the month: confinement and convalescence of Chinese women after childbirth. *Soc Sci Med.* 1978;2:11–22

13. Chung HJ. Understanding the oriental maternity patient. *Nurs Clin North Am.* 1977;12:67–75

14. Pang HC. Influence of the Chinese customs on the health-maintaining behaviors of the pregnant women. *J Veterans Hosp Taiwan.* 1993;10:247–251

15. Wexler-Morrison L, Anderson J, Richardson E. *Cross-Cultural Caring: A Handbook for Health Professionals.* Vancouver, BC: University of British Columbia Press; 1990

5
Perinatal Health Care Issues
of Cuban Women

Aleida Llanes-Oberstein

The US Bureau of the Census has projected that by 2010 the Hispanic-origin population may become the second-largest race/ethnic group in the United States.[1] In 2000 the Hispanic population in the United States was 32.8 million, or 12% of the total population; people of Cuban origin accounted for 4.0% of this figure,[2] with 68% living in the southern region of the United States.[3] By the year 2020 it is projected that the Cuban population will increase to 12.8 million, an increase of almost 2 million from 2001 data.[4] Approximately 71% of Cuban Americans were born in Cuba[5]; of these, the highest concentration (50%) reside in Miami, or "little Havana" as it is known.[6] Sizable Cuban colonies also exist in New Jersey, New York, California, Illinois, Texas, and Puerto Rico.[6]

Most Cubans immigrated to the United States during 3 distinct periods. In the years following the 1959 Cuban Revolution, several hundred thousand Cubans fled the island. This first large-scale immigration brought principally middle- and upper-class Cubans seeking political asylum.[4] Between 1959 and the conclusion of the 1980 Mariel boatlift, an estimated 1 million Cubans left the island permanently. This second wave of immigration brought a greater proportion of skilled, semiskilled, and unskilled workers.[4] During the mid-1990s an economic and political crisis sparked another mass exodus. As a humanitarian gesture, the United States instituted the Special Cuban Migration Program, or "Cuban lottery,"[7] through which a minimum of 20,000 Cubans would be issued travel documents each year and after a year become eligible to apply for US residency. In turn, Cuba pledged to discourage unsafe departures. However, some Cubans with valid US visas, physicians in particular, have been prohibited from leaving the island,[8] while Cuban refugees continue to take to the sea in alarming numbers.[9] Illegal immigration to the United States using homemade rafts, alien smugglers, or falsified visas continues. Approximately 3,000 Cubans attempted to cross the Florida straits in 2001, and only about 25% of these were intercepted by the US Coast Guard.[10]

This chapter will focus on those immigrant women whose degree of acculturation is minimal to none and whose state of health and beliefs continue to be greatly influenced by Cuba and the Cuban health care system.[11] In so doing, it must be underscored that changing food habits and styles of clothing, as well as learning and/or adapting to the majority language, tend to take place before the adoption of cultural beliefs, values, and more complex patterns of behavior.[12] Those women who immigrated soon after the revolution are no longer of childbearing age, but their grandmotherly influences will be discussed in the context of the Cuban family.

It would be shortsighted and possibly counterproductive to view Cuban women as newcomers who simply need to rapidly acculturate to American society. Latina immigrants bring with them certain cultural protections that serve to shield them from many high-risk health behaviors. These include steadfast support from family and friends, nutritious eating habits, positive attitudes toward motherhood and children, and low use of alcohol, tobacco, and illicit substances. Studies have documented that, regardless of socioeconomic status, health behaviors of Latinas worsen with increased levels of acculturation.[12–14] Thus an understanding of the demographics, customs, values, vital statistics, health care triumphs, and problems, as well as the culture's belief systems related to health, healing, and wellness, will enable health care providers to foster cultural practices that promote favorable health outcomes.

Cuba is an ethnically rich country with a population of 11.2 million (July 2002 estimate); 51% are mulatto, 37% white, 11% Afro-Cuban, and 1% Chinese. Racial intermingling is prominent throughout the island; 70% of the population are urban-based while 30% reside in rural settings.[10,15] The official language is Spanish, and the largest organized religion is Roman Catholic. Santería, a blend of beliefs and rituals brought to Cuba by African slaves, and Roman Catholicism, introduced by Spanish colonists, is also widely practiced. Protestants, Jehovah's Witnesses, and Jews account for a small segment of the population. Although Cuba has been an atheist state for most of the Castro era, the constitution was amended in 1992 to characterize the state as secular instead of atheist.

The 2002 estimated population data is as follows: Cuba's literacy rate (those aged 15 and older who can read and write) is 96.2% for males and 95.3% for females; the birth rate is 12.08 births per 1,000 and the death rate is 7.35 deaths per 1,000 population; life expectancy is 74.2 years for men and 79.15 years for women; and the total fertility rate is 1.6 children born per woman.[10,15,16] Women constitute 57% of the university graduates and 40% of the country's workforce.

Cubans have been described as highly individualistic people who are uninhibited emotionally. They tend to value *personalismo*, a person-oriented approach to social relations, and dislike impersonal relationships. Warmth, friendliness, hospitality, a strong sense of community, and a willingness to share what little they have are typical traits. *Simpatica* (charm) is highly valued. To be judged *antipático* or *pesado* (disagreeable) is anathema to them. To be *espléndido* (generous, giving) is another highly regarded trait. Frugality is not valued, and *tacañeria* (stinginess) is looked down on. Cubans have been described as fundamentally optimistic, persistent, and focused on the present. They are more likely to perceive work as necessary to attain a better, more enjoyable life, rather than as something of intrinsic value.[6] Their zest for life is often expressed through sensuality, gaiety, and loudness of voice.[4–6] They have a strong artistic presence and greatly enjoy music and dance.[17] *Relajo* (an attitude of freedom to do as one pleases) and humor are considered part of the traditional national character. *Choteo* (teasing) has helped Cubans endure life's unpleasantness. They exhibit a personal pride and self-confidence that can be misperceived as arrogance.

Of central importance to Cubans is the family, as is love for one's mother, paternal authority, and respect for older and deceased family members.[6] Pampering and babying of children are common, as are overprotection and a tendency to foster over-dependency. Cubans maintain close ties with the extended family, particularly during crisis periods, when relatives come together to offer support. Although Cuban workers are still paid in the national currency, the peso, some Cubans are able to supplement their incomes with US dollars sent to them by relatives in the United States, thereby helping to create 2 societies in Cuba—one with US dollars, the other without. Most new shops and food markets accept dollars only, not pesos.[18] Thus those who must rely exclusively on the peso and the food ration system are experiencing malnutrition. Women's health has been greatly affected by this dual currency. In a desperate search for US dollars from tourists, prostitution is on the rise along with sexually transmitted diseases (STDs).[19]

Health and Illness

In 1960 the Federation of Cuban Women (FCW) was established to put more women into the workplace and promote leadership roles for women. The organization now claims 3 million members, including 80% of women older than 14 years. Priorities of the FCW currently include maternal/infant health and family harmony, as well as issues related to the detection, education, and treatment of cervical and breast cancer. In addition, the FCW interfaces with psychiatrists, researchers, obstetrics and gynecology specialists, representatives from the Ministry of Public Health, and the media in activities to educate the community on issues of sexual health and the prevention of human immunodeficiency virus (HIV) and acquired immunodeficiency syndrome (AIDS). (Y.L. Marin, personal communication, 1997) Despite the fact that the life expectancy in Cuba has increased from 50 to 55 years (prerevolution) to the current 76.6 years, nutritional deficiencies began to emerge in the general population by 1993, as reflected in several health indices.[20–22] Most Cubans younger than 20 years have experienced a drop in their median weight. Children born in 1990 or later tend to be notably smaller than the same age group born in 1982. There has also been a sizable increase in the number of cases of osteoporosis in elderly women. This is primarily due to the inadequate supplies of calcium and calcium-rich foods. In addition, muscle and fat density as well as corporal mass have decreased for men and women between the ages of 20 and 60 years. Even though protein and caloric intake per capita has been on the rise since 1995, inequities remain in their consumption. Not all of the population is able to purchase food beyond that which is provided through rationed supplies, especially those who do not have access to US dollars. Unfortunately, the continued food and medicine shortage has further increased the incidence of malnutrition within the population.

With its emphasis on health promotion and disease prevention, Cuba's health care system has become an international model for primary and preventive health care. The family doctor-nurse team is the core of the primary health care model. No matter how simple or complex a health problem may be, the team continues to track, monitor, and visit the patient while communicating daily with any specialist that is on the case until the patient returns to the primary team. People are expected to use the health care system, and accommodations are made to encourage it. Parents are regularly given time off from work for their well-child doctor visits, their own checkups, prenatal care, and attendance at childbirth classes. A continuous health and medical record begins at birth and is maintained through death.

Children are encouraged to decorate and personalize their health journals. In addition to the community-based family doctor-nurse teams, there are teams in the workplace, clinics, schools, and other institutions to ensure continuity.

It is noteworthy that while infant mortality statistics from the 2000 Period Linked Birth/Infant Death Data Set revealed an overall infant mortality rate in the United States of 6.9 per 1,000 births, the rate for babies born to Cuban and Central and South American mothers combined (4.6) was lower than the rates for Puerto Rican (8.2) and Mexican (5.5) mothers.[15,23,24] Individually, Cuba registered an infant mortality rate of 6.4 deaths per 1,000 births in 1999, 7.2 deaths per 1,000 births in 2000, and 6.2 deaths per 1,000 births in 2001.[25,26] The 2001 estimated infant mortality rate for the United States was 6.4.[27]

Although great strides have been made in reducing the infant mortality rate in Cuba, maternal mortality continues to be a problem. The maternal mortality in 1999 was 43.8 deaths per 100,000 births, but decreased to 40.4 in 2000 and 33.9 in 2001[28]; 30% of the maternal deaths have been attributed to cesarean birth complications. Increased sepsis in the home and in the hospital, a lack of water supply, a lack of clean drinking water, antibiotic shortages, and poor nutritional status have all contributed to high morbidity and mortality among child-bearing women. The Ministry of Public Health has issued an alert and guidelines for reducing cesarean delivery birth rates from the current rates of 22% overall and 15% for primary cesarean deliveries.

Traditional and natural medicine has been fully integrated into the Cuban health care system. (L.P. Cacéres, personal interview, 1997). A Chinese medicine clinic offers acupuncture, massage, homeopathy, physiotherapy, tai chi, yoga, and *pelodoterapia* (mud therapy) for the management of hypertension, arthritis, asthma, anxiety, and depression. The homeopathic pharmacy or the green medicine department is an integral component of these treatment centers. The country is cultivating medicinal plants for the manufacture of "natural" pharmacology. Examples of such pharmaceuticals include an "energizer" for increasing libido and decreasing stress, garlic capsules as anti-inflammatories and analgesics, "sacred cane" for hypertension, fresh oregano heated in oil as ear drops for children, and oregano tinctures for colds. Acupuncture has been used for major surgery, as well as in the management of hyperemesis gravidarum, to stimulate breast milk production, for analgesia in laboring women, in the management of hyperbilirubinemia, and in the treatment of human papilloma virus, the premise being that acupuncture boosts the body's immune system.

Scientific rigor is very important to the Cubans. Research regarding the efficacy of every treatment modality is a national priority. Production of "medicinal" therapies is undertaken only after adequate clinical trials and under strict quality control. In 1996 47 million units of 100 different formulations of plant-based medicines were manufactured.[29,30] Each Cuban has access to using an average of 4.3 bottles of natural medicines per year, which is far below the demand. Cubans tend to continue using these herbal remedies even after immigrating to the United States; thus health care providers should elicit their usage when taking histories and be familiar with the most common ones. (See Table 5-1.)

Although the elimination of disparities between racial and ethnic groups is a major goal in Healthy People 2010,[36] the health indicators for Cubans in the United States are better than those of the other Hispanic subgroups. For example, Cubans have lower all-cause mortality rates (299.5 deaths per 100,000 births) than Puerto Ricans (406.1 deaths per 100,000 births) and Mexican Americans (348.4 deaths per 100,000 births).[37]

In 2000 Cuba had the highest percentage (21%) of those aged 65 and older, compared with 4.5% for Mexican and Central and South Americans; 41.3% of Cuban households consisted of only 2 people.[2] The disproportionate number of older people among Cubans stems

Table 5-1
Herbs Used by Cubans[29-35]

Botanical Name	English/Spanish Common Name	Condition Treated
Capsicum frutescens L.	Hot sauce (hot pepper)/Ají	Rheumatoid arthritis
Allium sativum L. (tincture and antiasthma syrup)*	Garlic/Ajo	Asthma, colds, improve circulation, hypertension
Ocimum basilcum L.	Sweet basil/Albahaca blanca	Stomachaches, hypertension
Indigofera suffruticosa M.	Añil de pasto/Añil cimarrón	Lice
Piper auritum H.B.K.	Vera cruz pepper/Caisimón de anis	Stomachaches, rheumatoid arthritis
Curcubita moschata D.	Spanish pumpkin/Calabaza	Parasites
Cassia grandis L.	Pink shower/Cañandonga	Fungal infections
Cymbopogon citratus D.C. (infusion)*	Sacred cane/Caña santa	Asthma, colds, sore throats, fungal infections, rheumatoid arthritis
Anethum graveolens B.	Dill/Eneldo	Stomachaches
Eucalyptus globulus L.	Tasmanian bluegupa or eucalyptus/Eucalipto	Asthma, colds, earaches, fever, coughs
Eucalyptus citriodora H.	Lemon scented gum/Eucalipto limo	Fever, coughs
Senna alata R.	Emperor's candlesticks/Guacamaya francesa	Fungal infections
Psidum guajaba L.	Guava/Guayaba	Diarrhea, fungal infections
Mentha spicata L.	Mint/Hierba buena	colds, intestinal gas
Foeniculum vulgare M.	Sweet fennel/Hinojo	Intestinal gas
Pedilanhtus tithymaloides L.	Jacob's ladder/Italmo real	Stomatitis, chancre sores
Jasminum officinale R.	Jasmine (5 leaves)/Jazmín de cinco hojas	Anxiety
Zingiber officinale R.	Garden ginger/Jengibre	Vomiting, coughs, intestinal gas
Citrus aurantifolia C.	Lemon/Limón	Improve circulation
Plantago major L.	Common plantain/Llantén mayor	Colds, stomatitis, chancre sores
Plantago lanceolata L.	Narrow leaf plantain/Llantén menor	Colds, burns, nasal congestion

Table 5-1
Herbs Used by Cubans[29-35]

Botanical Name	English/Spanish Common Name	Condition Treated
Matricaria recutita L. (tincture)†	Chamomille/Manzanilla	Diarrhea, stomachaches, fungal infections
Menta arvensis L.	Japanese mint/Menta japonesa	Stomachaches, intestinal gas
Murraya exotica L.	Orange jasmine/Muralla	Headaches
Citrus aurantium L.	Sour orange/Naranja agria	Improve circulation, stomachaches
Citrus sinensis L.	Sweet orange/Naranja dulce	Colds
Plectranthus amboinicus L.	French oregano/ Orégano francés	Colds, coughs
Passiflora incarnata	Purple passion flower/ Pasiflora	Anxiety
Mussa paradisiaca L.	Banana/Plátano	Lice
Lippia alba M.	Bushy matgrass/Quitadolor	Headaches
Ruta graveolens L.	Common rue/Ruda	Anxiety
Aloe barbadensis L.	Barbados aloe or aloe vera/Sábila	Asthma, colds, cuts, burns
Maranta arundinacea L.	Arrowroot/Sagú	Diarrhea
Salvia officinalis L. (syrup)*	Kitchen sage or common sage/Salvia de castilla	Colds, fungal infections, kidneys
Tamarindus indica L.	Tamarind/Tamarindo	Constipation, kidneys
Orthosiphon aristatus B.	Cat's whisker/Té de riñon	Diuretic
Justicia pectoralis J.‡	Freshcut/Tilo	Colds, anxiety
Melissa officinalis L.	Common balm or lemon balm/Toronjil	Diarrhea, fever
Menta piperita L.	Mint balm/Toronjil de menta	Colds, intestinal gas
Vetiveria zizanoides L.	Khuskhus vetiver/Vetiver	Fungal infections
Catharanthus roseus L.	Madagascar periwinkle/ Vicaria blanca	Conjunctivitis

*Do not administer to pregnant and lactating women.
†Do not administer to those in the first 5 months of pregnancy.
‡Do not administer to those on anticoagulants or individuals with clotting problems.

from the selective nature of their recent immigration. Due to their higher average age, Cubans have proportionately more people participating in the labor force, fewer unemployed individuals, and more workers at the peak of their earning power than the total US population.[6] Although 80% of Cubans have married, the divorce rate among those who have emigrated is quite high; 73% are high school graduates, and 23% have earned a bachelor's degree.[2] In 2000 5.8% of Cubans were unemployed; 34.4% earned $35,000 or more, which was the highest of the Latino subgroups; and 21% were reported to be uninsured.[2,12,38]

Although Cubans seem to have a strong health foundation, as immigrants they must overcome many obstacles. The loss of homeland, family separations, and lack of news from spouses, parents, or children who were unable to leave Cuba or who did not choose to do so often cause grief, anger, anxiety, or guilt.[6] Psychological scars caused by the avenue used to flee "the regime" are prominent, especially if the trip involved an illegal crossing of the Florida straits. Mental health problems such as anxiety and depression associated with immigration and relocation are common.[38] Poor economic conditions have resulted in micronutrient deficiencies in Cuban refugees, which, in turn, have been responsible for a recent epidemic of optic neuropathy, sensorineural deafness, peripheral sensory neuropathy, and dorsolateral myeloneuropathy.[39,40] Multivitamin supplements have curbed the epidemic, but health care providers should be alert to possible thiamine, cobalamin, folate, and sulfur amino acid deficits in Cuban refugees. Those that smoke are at highest risk (possibly because they lack adequate amounts of vitamins and minerals needed for cyanide detoxification) as are those who have inadequate intake of vitamin B_2, folate, or methionine. Open neural tube defects in infants may be increased due to folate deficiencies. Although the incidence of tuberculosis (TB) has been declining in Cuba since 1979, the age-adjusted prevalence for those born in Cuba (9.7%) is greater than those of Cuban descent who were born in the United States. Screening for sickle cell anemia is also important because of the high incidence of interracial marriage.[19] Dengue fever is another medical problem that has been identified among Cuban refugees. Thus hemoglobin or hematocrit testing, TB screening, and a nutritional assessment are recommended for Cuban refugees during their processing through immigration.[41,42]

For Cuban immigrants accustomed to the Cuban primary health care model of the family doctor-nurse team, accessing health services, even if they are insured, poses many challenges in the current managed care environment. These include difficulty getting appointments, lack of access to after-hours medical advice, and long waiting times for referrals to necessary medical specialists. Not only do Cuban women with limited English proficiency have difficulty with complex managed care enrollment and precertification practices for emergency room visits and hospitalizations, but they also face the hurdle of communicating with a provider who may not speak their language or value their cultural health beliefs and behaviors.[43,44] These obstacles can produce feelings of powerlessness.

While the uninsured rate for Hispanics was higher than for non-Hispanic whites, 35.3% versus 11.9% respectively,[45] Cuban women are more fortunate than other Hispanic immigrants because of unique immigration laws. Whether they immigrated by winning the "Cuban lottery" or sought political asylum by reaching US soil by some illegal route, Cubans are eligible for Medicaid, a nominal monthly stipend, a social security number, and a work permit as soon as they are processed by immigration. Once they find employment, however, the stipend and Medicaid coverage ends.[46]

The family doctor-nurse team in Cuba establishes a personalized patient-physician relationship that is based on mutual understanding and trust, allowing open discussions of health care concerns and problems.[47] There have been reports that Latin Americans distrust the US health care system, with 27% believing that they experience discrimination in gaining access to quality services and 30% believing they are not treated with respect.[48] To a culture that expects intense, personal contact from providers, the conventional Western distancing behavior can seem cold and uncaring. Family members have a prominent role in decisions regarding health care. When Cubans are hospitalized in a Cuban hospital, there is always a family member with them 24 hours a day regardless of the age of the patient.

Latin Americans develop *confianza* (confidence, trust) in their health care providers after a relationship has been established, unlike many Americans who exhibit confidence in their provider early on in the relationship.[49] *Respeto* is an expectation of deference and respect for an individual's age, gender, or position of authority. Although Cubans generally use the informal tense when speaking, health care providers can convey respect by using the formal tense when speaking Spanish, providing eye contact, speaking in a polite manner, and permitting the participation of the head of the household (often the spouse or grandparent).[5,50] Out of respect for the provider's position of authority, Hispanics often refrain from expressing disagreement or even asking questions, regardless of what they may be thinking. Health care providers who do not speak Spanish should use a "cultural" interpreter who thoroughly understands the Cuban culture. They should also make an attempt to speak even a few words or phrases in Spanish, which will lower barriers and invite trust.[51] Familiarity with such common concerns as *mal de ojo* (evil eye), *empacho* (indigestion), *decaimiento* (lack of energy), *desmayo* (fainting spells), and *barrenillos* (obsessive thinking)[6,52] will also convey cultural sensitivity, as will an awareness of Cuban food preferences. (See Table 5-2.)

The incidence of Santería among Cubans in the United States is unknown; however, it is said to be widespread, having proliferated to an extent beyond that previously achieved in Cuba.[6,56] Central to Santería is a belief in the dual nature of humans (ie, a separation of body and soul). *Santos* (saints) are viewed as having the same propensity toward

Table 5-2
Cuban Food Choices[53-55]

Protein	Dairy	Grains	Vegetables	Fruits	Fats & Oils	Other
Red snapper	Cow milk	White rice—	Olives	Pineapples	Olive oil	Seasonings
Crab	Goat milk	enriched	Avocado	Guavas	Lard	Garlic
Shrimp	Cheese	Macaroni	Chayote	Papayas	Vegetable oil	Salt
Lobster	Yogurt	Wheat flour	Red peppers	(fruta bomba)	Coconut oil	Pepper
Salted cod	Condensed milk	Corn meal	Asparagus	Bananas	Butter	Cooking wine
(bacalao)	Evaporated milk	Noodles	Okra	Coconuts	Corn oil	Vinegar
Squid	Ice cream	Spaghetti	(quimbombo)	Oranges		Onion
Clams			Spanish pumpkin	Lemons		Mustard
Oysters			Lettuce	Limes		Cumin
Mussels			Tomatoes	Grapefruits		Saffron
Sword fish			Eggplant	Tamarinds		Sugar
Sardines			Raddishes	Mangoes		Honey
Chicken			Cabbage	Mamay		Tomato sauce
Duck			Plantain	Prunes		Mayonnaise
Turkey			Sweet potatoes	Plums		Ketchup
Pork			Corn (tamal)	Dates		Snacks
Beef			Watercress	Figs		Peanuts
Veal			Carrots	Strawberries		Cashews
Goat			Beets	Apples		Almonds
Soy			Celery	Peaches		Fruit
Eggs			Cucumbers	Melons		Ice cream
Black beans			String beans	Raisins		Cookies

Table 5-2
Cuban Food Choices[53-55], continued

Protein	Dairy	Grains	Vegetables	Fruits	Fats & Oils	Other
Chick peas			Onions	Grapes		Crackers
Lentils			Potatoes	Cherries		Bread sticks
Split peas			Malanga	Pears		Coffee
Black-eyed peas			Yuca	Sugar cane		Espresso
Red kidney						
beans						
Lima beans						

good and evil as humans.[4] Today Santería is used primarily for dealing with personal crises and spiritual and emotional problems. It reduces feelings of despondency and helplessness. It gives Cubans protection in a chaotic world. It contributes to an improved sense of mastery over one's life. It also reduces uncertainty in life and alleviates certain physical conditions.

Pregnancy/Prenatal Care

Cuban women have the lowest fertility rate of all racial and ethnic groups in the United States and are most likely to have their children between the ages of 25 and 29 years.[23] Although pregnancy is viewed by Cubans as a normal, physiologic event, childbearing families in Cuba receive special attention and protection within the Constitution, Family Code, and labor laws. For example, mothers-to-be are eligible for paid maternity leave for 6 months, with an additional 6 months of optional leave without pay; fathers-to-be get 1 week off with pay to attend childbirth preparation. Day care at the workplace *(Circulo Infantil)* is provided. A nominal fee for child care covers food and the washing of children's clothes, and a law reserves the front seats of public buses for pregnant women. If there is concern over a pregnant woman's inadequate weight gain, supplemental meals will be provided in her workplace. If a pregnancy is determined to be high risk, the woman is housed in a beautiful and spotless maternity home that is staffed with nurses and an obstetrician, presented with many educational offerings, given ample opportunity to rest, and nourished well. During her confinement, the community is obliged to take care of her home and family. Pregnant women rely greatly on their mothers and grandmothers for advice and support during the pregnancy, birth, and postpartum period.[51] However, the traditional support of extended family so central to Cuban culture might be absent or severely limited following immigration to the United States. For a new, inexperienced mother this loss is profound, making an already stressful transition to a new country even more difficult.[49]

In 2001 91.9% of Cuban mothers who gave birth in the United States began prenatal care in the first trimester.[27,57] The more highly educated[58] tend to be receptive to routine blood testing, sonography, and screening for STDs, HIV, AIDs, sickle cell anemia, and TB because these tests are routinely done in Cuba. Nutritional assessments and counseling early in the prenatal course are critical, especially for younger Cuban Americans who tend to have higher total and saturated fat and lower carbohydrate intakes than older Cubans and other Hispanic subgroups living in the United States.[21,58,59] In addition, food shortages in Cuba have resulted in micronutrient deficiencies among many pregnant Cuban immigrants.[59] However, they tend to have the lowest rate of anemia during pregnancy, compared with other Hispanics, whites, and blacks,[23] even though anemia remains a problem in Cuba. The use of herbs during pregnancy is also prevalent.

Even though there is a high incidence of tobacco exposure among Cubans, and until recently, cigarettes were included in the ration basket, tobacco use during pregnancy among women of Cuban origin in 2000 was only 3.3%, much lower than other Hispanics, whites, and blacks.[27,57] However, there does seem to be a correlation between acculturation and alcohol consumption among Cuban American women.[38,60]

In the United States, pregnancy-induced hypertension is responsible for approximately one third of the pregnancy-related deaths of Hispanic women.[20] Additionally, Hispanics living in the United States are almost twice as likely to die from diabetes as are non-Hispanic whites[36]; in recognition of this, the US Department of Health and Human Services established an objective of reducing diabetes among this population in Healthy People 2000 and 2010.[36,55,57]

A 77.5% incidence of STDs was reported among 120 pregnant women who participated in a Havana study in 1997.[61] Thus it is important to screen for STDs among all immigrant Cuban woman. From 1996 through 1999, 2,299 tested positive for HIV (24.9% were women); heterosexual transmission accounted for 41.1% of the cases.[62] By November 2001, 5 months after the Cuban public health system introduced domestically manufactured antiretrovirals for patients with AIDS, deaths from AIDS and the incidence of opportunistic infections among patients with HIV and AIDS registered a decrease from the same period 1 year before.[63] Today HIV testing of all pregnant women in Cuba is mandatory.

There is much folklore surrounding pregnancy that tends to be held by the less educated Cubans.[61] (A. Collazo and Z. de la Nuez, personal interview, 1997). (See Table 5-3.) One folk belief is that a pregnant woman should obey any cravings (*antojos*) she may have for specific foods or the baby may be born with characteristics of the particular food; for example, a hemangioma may be present if the mother craves strawberries but does not consume them.[57] Many believe that a mother who looks at a handicapped child during her pregnancy will birth an infant with the same handicap. Still another folk belief is *caida de mollera* (fallen fontanel), which is believed to be caused by holding or picking up a baby improperly, moving or carrying it roughly, bouncing it while playing, or separating it from the mother's breast too quickly.[57] The Afro-Cuban religion of Santería further teaches that when babies come into the world, they are accompanied by an *Orisha*, which is thought to be one of their first lines of protection in life. The baby shares many of the traits of the *Orisha;* thus knowing the "owner of one's head" helps them to know themselves better and to lead more effective lives. The more they live in harmony with their *Orisha,* the more harmonious their lives will be.[56]

Labor and Delivery

Cuban immigrant women compare favorably with other Latinas, whites, and African Americans in terms of medical risk factors, complications, and obstetric interventions; dysfunctional labors and cesarean births are 2 exceptions. (See Table 5-4.) The Centers for Disease Control and Prevention reports that the cesarean birth rate

Table 5-3
Pregnancy- and Newborn-Related Beliefs/Folklore

Practice or Symptom	Belief
Heartburn.	Baby will have a lot of hair.
Pregnant woman looks at a lunar eclipse.	Baby will have a pigmented birth mark on the face.
Wearing necklaces during pregnancy.	A nuchal cord might result.
Buying crib before the baby is born.	Bad luck will follow.
"Aantojos" (food cravings).	A pregnant woman should be given what she craves; if not, the baby will be born with its mouth opened.
Ear piercing of baby girls; usually done in the hospital before discharge.	
40 days postpartum: sexual abstinence.	Sexual intercourse can cause postpartum psychosis.
Consumption of "Orchata" malt (almond cream blended with milk).	Milk supply will increase.
No one should drink from a breastfeeding mother's glass.	Must not "steal" the mother's milk.
A breastfeeding mother should not be upset.	Breast milk will be bad for the baby.
Baby should not be exposed to light from the moon while sleeping.	Baby could die.
A protruding umbilical stump should be reduced by a belly band until cord falls off.	Umbilical hernia can be avoided.
Put a wet thread on a hiccupping baby's forehead.	Hiccups will stop.
When a baby has a high fever, put a salvia leaf with lard and coffee on the soles of the baby's feet and cover with a sock; rub Albaca over the baby's body.	The fever will subside.
Give a colicky baby a teaspoon of coconut "grease."	Colic will subside.
Don't touch fontanels.	Baby can die.
"Azabache" (black Carribean stone) with a red ribbon should be placed on the baby	To ward off the "evil eye."

Table 5-3
Pregnancy- and Newborn-Related Beliefs/Folklore

Practice or Symptom	Belief
Mother becomes more beautiful during the pregnancy.	The baby will be a girl.
Mother not attractive during the pregnancy.	The baby will be a boy.
Put 2 chairs next to each other; place a scissor on one and a knife on the other.	If the pregnant woman sits on the scissor, the baby will be a girl; if she sits on the knife, the baby will be a boy.
Children and adults should be kissed on the cheek, never on the lips; babies should be kissed on the forehead.	Baby may become infected; kissing on the lips is reserved for lovers.
Other women's health-related beliefs If women wash their hair during menses.	Menstrual flow will stop.
Masturbation by adolescents.	Causes psychosis.

for Cuban women living in the United States is nearly 50% higher than those for any other population subgroup.[64] The reason for this perplexing statistic is unclear. However, Cuban babies had the lowest percentage of 5-minute Apgar scores below 7 (0.8%) than any other group in 2000.[27] (See Table 5-5.)

Natural childbirth is preferred by Cuban women. More and more are enrolling in childbirth classes with their partners because attendance is greatly encouraged in Cuba. Fathers are becoming more involved in decision making, but grandmothers continue to play a primary role. More fathers are attending the birth process, but usually as an observer and always in addition to the grandmother or other female support person. Cuban women are very modest and appreciate respect for their privacy. Typically children are not present at the birth.

Pharmacologic analgesia and anesthesia are generally not favored in Cuba. Acupuncture may provide pain relief during labor for some

Table 5-4
Number and Rate of Live Births to Mothers With Selected Medical Risk Factors, Complications of Labor, and Obstetric Procedures by Hispanic Origin of Mother and Race for Mothers of Non-Hispanic Origin, United States 2000 (per 1,000 live births)

Medical Risk Factors, Complications, and Obstetric Procedures	All Origins	Total Hispanic	Mexican	Puerto Rican	Cuban	Central and South American	Other and Unknown	Total Non-Hispanic	White	Black
Anemia	23.9	24.5	23.3	36.4	18.3	17.2	42.9	23.7	20.0	37.7
Diabetes	29.3	28.3	27.3	36.6	24.4	29.4	29.7	29.5	28.3	27.3
Hypertension, pregnancy-associated	38.8	27.9	27.0	31.6	31.7	27.2	35.3	41.7	43.2	41.9
Uterine bleeding	6.6	4.2	3.9	6.6	2.4	3.9	5.9	7.0	7.4	5.7
Meconium, moderate/heavy	53.9	58.9	58.0	58.4	40.3	65.6	60.6	52.6	47.2	72.2
Premature rupture of membranes	24.6	17.8	15.6	28.5	19.4	19.7	26.1	26.1	25.4	29.3
Dysfunctional labor	28.2	24.2	20.6	33.9	40.4	30.5	36.3	29.0	29.4	25.6
Breech/malpresentation	38.8	30.4	28.5	39.5	37.7	32.6	34.7	40.8	44.0	30.6
Cephalopelvic disproportion	17.2	13.2	13.2	14.0	13.7	13.3	12.2	18.3	19.4	12.9
Fetal distress	39.2	30.4	27.8	40.3	26.7	34.3	35.3	41.1	39.5	48.8
Amniocentesis	24.0	11.1	7.9	19.3	24.4	18.8	18.3	27.2	29.7	15.4
Electronic fetal monitoring	842.0	798.2	785.6	869.1	867.6	805.2	829.2	853.7	859.1	851.3
Induction of labor	198.8	131.6	124.2	159.8	184.6	127.6	180.9	215.6	235.6	164.6
Ultrasound	670.0	583.5	562.4	683.6	601.5	607.1	658.1	692.0	716.9	608.6
Stimulation of labor	179.5	166.4	160.1	212.9	171.5	175.4	164.2	182.8	187.3	164.6

Table 5-5
Percentage of Births With Selected Medical or Health Characteristics by Origin, Race, and Place of Birth of Mother, United States 2000[27]

Characteristics	All Origins	Maternal Hispanic Origin						Non-Hispanic		
		Total	Mexican	Puerto Rican	Cuban	Central and South American	Other & Unknown	Total	White	Black
All Births: Infants	Rate									
Preterm births	11.6	11.2	11.0	13.5	10.6	11.0	12.2	11.7	10.4	17.4
Birthweight										
birthweight of <1,500 g	1.4	1.1	1.0	1.9	1.2	1.2	1.4	1.5	1.1	3.1
birthweight of <2,500 g	7.6	6.4	6.0	9.3	6.5	6.3	7.8	7.9	6.6	13.1
birthweight of ≥4,000 g	9.9	9.0	9.3	7.3	9.5	9.0	7.4	10.1	11.7	5.3
5-minute Apgar score of <7	1.4	1.1	1.2	1.4	0.8	1.0	1.2	1.4	1.2	2.4
Births to mothers born in the 50 states and DC										
Preterm births	11.9	12.1	11.9	13.5	10.5	10.9	12.7	11.9	10.5	17.8
Birthweight										
birthweight of <1,500 g	1.5	1.3	1.2	2.0	1.1	1.2	1.4	1.5	1.1	3.1
birthweight of <2,500 g	7.9	7.3	6.8	9.2	6.5	7.1	8.3	7.9	6.6	13.5
birthweight of ≥4,000 g	10.2	8.2	8.6	7.4	8.4	8.6	7.1	10.4	11.7	5.0
5-minute Apgar score of <7	1.4	1.3	1.3	1.4	0.8	1.0	1.3	1.5	1.2	2.4

Table 5-5
Percentage of Births With Selected Medical or Health Characteristics by Origin, Race, and Place of Birth of Mother, United States 2000[27]

Characteristics	All Origins	Maternal Hispanic Origin							Non-Hispanic		
		Total	Mexican	Puerto Rican	Cuban	Central and South American	Other & Unknown	Total	White	Black
Births to mothers born outside the 50 states and DC										
Preterm births	10.5	10.7	10.5	13.5	10.8	11.0	10.5	10.2	9.1	14.0
Birthweight										
birthweight of <1,500 g	1.1	1.0	0.9	1.9	1.3	1.2	1.1	1.2	0.9	2.6
birthweight of <2,500 g	6.4	5.8	5.5	9.4	6.5	6.3	6.0	7.1	5.8	9.8
birthweight of ≥4,000 g	8.9	9.5	9.8	7.0	10.3	9.1	8.5	8.1	11.3	8.3
5-minute Apgar score of <7	1.1	1.1	1.1	1.5	0.8	1.0	0.8	1.2	0.9	2.0

while local anesthetics are used for the repair of episiotomies and lac-erations. Electronic fetal monitoring and intravenous hydration are used only when indicated. Auscultation of the fetal heart with a feto-scope is routine. Hospital births are perceived to correlate with low infant and maternal mortality; thus the Cuban immigrant generally avoids out-of-hospital birth settings.

In Cuba, the woman assumes positions of her choice during labor. The upright position and ambulation are highly encouraged. Labor and birth units have squatting bars in the labor rooms to be used dur-ing the second stage of labor. Eating and drinking are also encouraged during labor, and the family provides the nourishment. Women tend to be stoic during birth, but are not discouraged from being expres-sive. The poor economic conditions in Cuba have prevented renova-tions of most maternity hospitals; thus births occur in prerevolution 1950s delivery rooms with the woman in the lithotomy position. Mediolateral episiotomies are plentiful, especially in first-time moth-ers. Some obstetric practitioners continue an old practice of routinely suturing the cervix at "3 and 9 o'clock," ostensibly to "decrease the incidence of cervical cancer"; thus cervical scarring is common in multiparous Cuban women.

Cuban hospitals never separate the mother and infant after the birth unless medically necessary. Breastfeeding is initiated in the deliv-ery room. The mother is taken from the delivery room to the recovery room in a wheelchair carrying her baby. The recovery room is staffed by a pediatrician and neonatal nurse. The baby is examined at the mother's bedside; once both are stable, they are transferred to the postpartum unit. All mothers have rooming-in. Central nurseries are used as storage rooms. Mothers with babies in the neonatal intensive care unit are very involved in the infant's care.

The support of female family members, encouragement and as-surances from health care providers that "everything is normal," and demonstrations of love and affection from her spouse or partner are very important to the Cuban immigrant woman during labor and birth. Programs that use *comadres* (community workers who support women during the perinatal period) and institutions that provide midwifery services are accepted within Latino communities.[57]

Postpartum and Newborn Care

A 40-day recovery period, known as *la cuarentena,* is observed by new mothers in Cuba. The grandmothers and other female members of the extended family generally take care of the infant, mother, and housework.[57] Breastfeeding and taking care of the infant are the new mother's priorities. Sexual intercourse is avoided during this 40-day period. Girdles are believed to aid in involution and improving abdominal muscle tone and are commonly used.

Circumcision is not performed. First-born children are typically named after their parents. Both parents' surnames are used with the father's preceding the mother's. An infant born on a saint's day may be named after that saint. Infants are typically carried. Infant carriers and strollers are not encouraged.

Binding of the baby's umbilicus after birth is preferred by many Cuban mothers to the usually recommended air-drying of the umbilical stump. Its purpose is to prevent bulging or herniation around the umbilicus and also to "keep the intestines from falling out." Many of the binders *(fajeros)* are elaborately decorated with fine embroidery and other ornamental items and are given as gifts for the new baby. Infections or other skin irritations are seldom observed in babies who have had the binding, but on occasion an omphalitis can develop. Respect for the practice can be balanced with friendly advice to keep the binding relatively loose and to use *fajeros* made of cotton.[57]

Determined to make breastfeeding a national priority, education in Cuba begins with the youngest of children. One nationally popular cartoon character charges the bottle with his sword, sending the message that cow milk is not for babies. Support for breastfeeding is further reinforced throughout the school years, in the workplace, and during prenatal care. (M.T. Esperson, personal interview, 1997). Cuba has succeeded in making every maternity hospital a UNICEF mother- and baby-friendly hospital and in achieving successful lactation in greater than 95% of women on discharge postpartum. In the postpartum areas, not a bottle of formula can be found; mothers and babies room together and do not leave the hospital until lactation is established. The only exceptions are HIV carriers, for whom supplements in the form of breast milk from other lactating women are made available. At 4 months postpartum, 50% of urban and 70% of rural women are still breastfeeding their babies; in some municipalities that number reaches as high as 94%. Unfortunately, nursing rates begin to decline when Cuban immigrants are confronted by the many formula choices in the United States and are given ready-to-use formula on discharge from the hospital. This is a prime example when health care providers can support the successes of the country of origin. Cuban immigrant women need encouragement in withstanding the temptations to bottle-feed. A bilingual lay mentor or a doula, preferably Cuban, may also be needed to assist with breastfeeding postpartum.[47]

Cubans often believe that the mother is culpable when a child is born with a genetic defect such as Down syndrome. The mother is blamed for not taking care of herself. The genetic defect can be attributed to past sins. Thus the punishment is carried out on the child. If the child is severely disabled, then he or she typically will be taken care of in the home, with the women of the household taking responsibility.[4]

Family Planning

In Cuba, a couple's individual choice regarding the size and timing of their families prevails. Until 1990 Cuban women relied on birth control pills as their primary means of contraception. The embargo led to a drastic reduction of pills imported from various places and irregularity in the types of pills obtained. As a result, women were being switched from 1 type of pill to another, which led to fluctuating hormone levels and a very dissatisfying experience. Barrier methods are equally scarce. Condoms are not easily acquired. The diaphragm would not be a desirable method for Cuban women, even if available, and contraceptive creams or jellies are virtually nonexistent.[22] At present, the intrauterine device (IUD) is the most commonly used method in Cuba. This brings an increased risk of ectopic pregnancies and pelvic inflammatory disease to a health care system that is already compromised because of limited medications and supplies. The situation is further exacerbated by the lack of adequate supplies of antibiotics for early treatment. Cuban immigrant women tend to prefer hormonal contraceptives and IUDs.

The participation of Cuban males in the family planning process continues to be a problem. A Cuban study reported that only 8% of adolescents used any form of contraception in their first sexual experience and only 26% were currently using contraception. The main reason given for not using condoms was reduced sensation perceived during intercourse.[65]

Cuban women achieved the right to quality abortion services in the early 1960s as part of their struggle for full gender equality and in response to the increased maternal mortality and high incidence of mutilations, which resulted from the extensive and indiscriminate practice of illegal abortions. The time limit for abortions by choice in Cuba is 10 weeks after the last menstrual period.[66] Although it is estimated that 25% of the abortions performed in Cuba are directly related to contraceptive failure, some women rely on pregnancy termination as a means of contraception.[21] More than half of those seeking abortions do so outside of their community of residence because of a lingering stigma.[59,67]

Recent Cuban immigrants in the United States tend to identify themselves as "prochoice." However, with the availability of a variety of contraceptive options available to them, they are less likely to rely on abortion as a means of contraception.

Bioethical Dilemmas

The high divorce rate among Cuban immigrants has been attributed to dramatic shifts in roles experienced by Cuban immigrants. Many women who would be full-time homemakers in their native land must now work outside the home to provide needed income while continuing to bear the burdens of housekeeping and child rearing, which are not part of the *machista's* roles.[6] Although Cuban fathers are being encouraged to take a more active role in pregnancy-related issues, their machismo ideals and their traditional roles of sole provider and disciplinarian are in direct conflict with such involvement. As Cuban women receive less attention from their husbands, they turn their energies and attentions to their unborn babies and older children[4]; such devotion can thus be viewed as compensatory and not dysfunctional.

Among Cuban American women, higher levels of acculturation have been correlated with a history of multiple sex partners. This trend is of concern because Hispanic males have reported a high incidence of unprotected sex and a low perceived risk of HIV infection, placing Latina women at an ever-increasing risk for HIV transmission through vaginal sex.[38] One Cuban study reported that 61% of the young male participants did not acknowledge their responsibility for contraception and believed that they were well within their rights in demanding unprotected sex from their partners[65]; this has been attributed to that machista (sexist) attitudes.

Counseling regarding the cause of an infant's illness or congenital anomaly is also challenging because the Cuban woman may think that she is being punished for past sins or that during her pregnancy she looked at another child with the same anomaly. Or, a visible anomaly such as a cleft lip may be blamed on a nonmedical cause such as *brujería* (witchcraft). Other Cuban American families may accept the anomaly as part of a larger divine plan designed by God to make them better parents. In some instances, it is seen as a blessing to be the parents of a special child. Family members who hold these beliefs may be less open to using the services of a health care professional.

Religious and folk beliefs are deeply ingrained in Cuban culture. The supernatural is often held responsible for illnesses and their cures, while diagnosis and treatment by a health care provider are viewed as supplementary. Problems that a health care provider might regard as needing medical intervention may instead be perceived by the woman as spiritual. When the woman has also sought the advice of a priest, *santero* or *santera* (faith or folk healer), collaboration is generally beneficial but may present an ethical dilemma for the provider.[6,52] Because some women believe that "invisible" medical conditions do not exist, it is extremely challenging to help women see that an invisible condition, such as an asymptomatic urinary tract infection, requires treatment in spite of the fact that she may feel fine.[4]

Terminally ill Cuban babies are traditionally given the last rites. Non-Christian health care providers must be sensitive to the importance of the last rites and be familiar with what administering them entails. They may be called on by the family to administer the last rites if a priest is not readily available.

Death/Burial Rites

A perinatal death is a family tragedy. When faced with a pregnancy loss, women/couples are supported by their extended families. Their strong belief in their faith guides them through this difficult time. Acceptance is made easier by the belief that "it was the will of God" or the Cuban fatalistic sense that events are determined by forces outside of one's control.[5,6] The deceased infant is named and is believed to have ascended into heaven. In Cuba, the overnight wake typically occurs in the home. Burial occurs the following morning. It is suggested that family members be included in bereavement counseling whenever possible. Family therapy is often the treatment of choice.

Every Cuban Woman is Unique

Cuban women immigrate to the United States with a solid foundation of primary preventive health care. They are deeply rooted in Cuban traditions and love their homeland. Health care providers must help them in culturally sensitive ways to undergo a smooth transition to their new land while supporting the positive health behaviors they derived from Cuba. Mutual *respeto* and *confianza* provide the underpinnings for effective perinatal health care for clients of Cuban origin.

Perinatal Health Care Issues of Cuban Women: Key Highlights

Demographic/Psychosocial/Spiritual Characteristics

- In 2000 people of Cuban origin comprised 4.0% of the Hispanic population in the United States.
- Cuba is an ethnically rich country comprised of 51% mulatto, 37% white, 11% Afro-Cuban, and 1% Chinese.
- The official language is Spanish. Health care workers who speak Spanish and understand Cuban culture facilitate health care services.
- Cuba's literacy rate is 95.3% for females and 96.2% for males.
- The life expectancy is 79.15 years for women and 74.2 years for men.
- Women constitute 57% of the university graduates and 40% of the workforce.
- The fertility rate is 1.6 children per woman.
- Women show respect by being compliant, very polite, and not questioning the provider.
- Eye contact is considered a sign of respect.
- Cubans present a mixture of informality, individualism, and deference in interpersonal relationships
- Charm and generosity are highly valued.
- There is a tendency to speak quickly and loudly.

- Hugging and kissing on the cheek are part of the typical greeting.
- Depression and psychological scars from family separation and memories of traumatic exits from Cuba may be exhibited.
- A female attendant is preferred; most physicians in Cuba are female.
- The largest organized religion is Roman Catholic.
- Afro-Cuban religions (Santería) are widely practiced.
- Smaller numbers of Protestants, Jehovah's Witnesses, and Jews are represented.

Prenatal Care
- In Cuba, women receive early and comprehensive prenatal care.
- Pregnancy-induced hypertension is the leading cause of pregnancy-related deaths among Cubans.
- Cubans living in the United States are twice as likely to die from diabetes as are non-Hispanic whites.
- Malnutrition is common; pregnant women should be screened for folate deficiency, anemia, and intrauterine growth restriction.

Prenatal Testing
- Sonographies are accepted.
- Routine prenatal blood testing and screening for STDs, HIV, AIDs, sickle cell anemia, diabetes, and TB are important and accepted.
- Women and their partners are usually amenable to genetic counseling and testing.

Pregnancy Diet
- Multivitamin supplementation is recommended due to micronutrient deficiencies.
- If available, beef, pork, poultry, fish, and legumes are preferred protein sources; soy is being used as an alternative.

Pregnancy-Related Beliefs/Taboos
- See Table 5-3.

Labor and Delivery

- Natural childbirth is preferred.
- While pharmacologic pain relief is generally avoided, acupuncture may be used for analgesia and anesthesia; local anesthesia is used for the repair of episiotomies and lacerations.
- Electronic fetal monitoring and intravenous hydration are used only when indicated; fetal heart auscultation with a fetoscope is routine.
- More than 95% of births occur in the hospital.
- Women assume positions of choice during labor. The upright position, ambulation, and squatting are highly encouraged.
- Eating and drinking is encouraged during labor; the family provides the nourishment.
- A family member is always present for support; typically it is the woman's mother or other female relative. Fathers do participate, but usually as observers.
- Women tend to be stoic during birth, but are not discouraged from being expressive.

Postpartum Care

- A 40-day recovery period *(la cuarentena)* is observed.
- Breastfeeding and taking care of the infant are the mother's priorities; housework is done by extended family.
- Sexual intercourse is avoided during the 40-day period.
- Girdles are commonly used; it is believed that they aid in involution and improving abdominal muscle tone.

Postpartum Diet

- See Pregnancy Diet.

Neonatal Care

- Circumcision is not performed.
- First-born children are typically named after their parents; both parents' surnames are used, the father's followed by the mother's.
- An infant born on a saint's day may be named after that saint.
- Infants are typically carried.
- Mothers and babies are never separated from the time of birth unless medically necessary.
- Beliefs about infants with illness or congenital anomalies are often attributed to external forces.
- Binding of the baby's umbilicus after birth is a frequently observed custom.

Breastfeeding/Breast Care

- The benefits of breastfeeding are understood, making it the preferred method in Cuba.
- In the United States, Cuban immigrants need support and encouragement to resist the lures of advertisements and gift packages that promote bottle-feeding.
- A balanced diet is very important to increase milk supply.

Family Planning

- Male contraception is not acceptable due to machismo.
- Oral contraceptives and IUDs are preferred.
- The diaphragm is not a desirable method.
- Surgical sterilizations are acceptable.
- Small families are preferred.

Family Involvement

- While fathers are becoming more involved in decision making, grandmothers continue to play a main role.
- More fathers are attending the birth process, but usually in addition to the grandmother or other female support person.
- Other children are not present at the birth.

- Grandmothers and other female members of the extended family participate in early infant care and care of the mother.

Pregnancy Termination/Miscarriage

- Abortion is accepted for pregnancy problems and contraceptive failures.

Bioethical Dilemmas

- Some believe that "invisible" medical conditions do not exist and do not warrant investigation or treatment.
- Congenital anomalies may be interpreted as punishment for past sins.
- Medical problems may be regarded as spiritual. The woman may seek advice from a priest or faith or folk healer.

Death/Burial Rites

- A perinatal death is a family tragedy.
- A stillborn infant is named.
- In Cuba, an overnight viewing typically occurs in the home; burial occurs the following morning.

References

1. US Department of Commerce, Bureau of the Census. *Profile of the Hispanic Population in the United States.* Washington, DC: US Government Printing Office; 2000. PPL 136
2. US Department of Commerce, Bureau of the Census. *The Hispanic Population in the United States: Population Characteristics.* Washington, DC: US Government Printing Office; 2001
3. Centers for Disease Control and Prevention. Health outcomes among Hispanic subgroups: data from the National Health Interview Survey, 1992-95. *Advance Data.* 2000;310:1–15
4. Brice A. *An Introduction to Cuban Culture for Rehabilitation Service Providers.* Buffalo, NY: Center for International Rehabilitation Research Information Exchange University at Buffalo State University of New York; 2002. Available at: http://cirrie.buffalo.edu/cuba.html. Accessed February 1, 2003
5. Huff RM, Kline MV. *Promoting Health in Multicultural Populations: A Handbook for Practitioners.* London, UK: Sage Publications; 1999

6. Gueralt M. Understanding Cuban immigrants: a cultural perspective. *Social Work.* 1984;29:115–121

7. US Department of State. *Fact Sheet: The Cuban Adjustment Act.* Available at: http://www.state.gov/www/regions/wha/cuba/cuba_adjustment_act.html. Accessed February 1, 2003

8. Stout D. US says Cuba causes misery with its hard line on emigres. *New York Times.* August 29, 2000:A8

9. US Department of State. *Cuba: Migration.* Available at: http://www.state.gov/www/regions/wha/cuba/migration.html. Accessed February 1, 2003

10. US Department of State. *Cuba: Country Information.* Available at: http://www.state.gov/www/regions/wha/cuba/country_info.html. Accessed February 1, 2003

11. Rew L. Access to health care for Latina adolescents: a critical review. *J Adol Health.* 1998;23:194–204

12. Aguirre-Molina M, Molina CW, Zambrana RE, eds. *Health Issues in the Latino Community.* San Francisco, CA: Jossey-Bass; 2001

13. Abraido-Lanza AF, Dohrenwend BP, Ng-Mak DS, Turner JB. The Latino mortality paradox: a test of the 'salmon bias' and healthy migrant hypotheses. *Am J Public Health.* 1999;89:1543–1548

14. Cohen E, Goode TD. *Rationale for Cultural Competence in Primary Health Care.* Washington, DC: National Center for Cultural Competence; 1999

15. US Central Intelligence Agency. *The World Factbook 2002—Cuba.* Available at: http://www.odci.gov/cia/publications/factbook/geos/cu.html. Accessed February 1, 2003

16. ABC News. *Country Profile: Cuba.* Available at: http://www.abcnews.go.com/reference/countries/CU.html. Accessed February 1, 2003

17. *The Cuban experience: Culture.* Available at: http://www.library.thinkquest.org/18355/culture.html. Accessed February 1, 2003

18. Putman JJ. Evolution in the revolution: Cuba. *National Geographic.* 1999;195:2–45

19. Barry M. Effect of the US embargo and economic decline on health in Cuba. *Ann Intern Med.* 2000;132:151–154

20. Bureau of Inter-American Affairs. *Zenith and Eclipse: A Comparative Look at Socio-Economic Conditions in Pre-Castro and Present Day Cuba, 1998.* Available at: http://www.state.gov/www/regions/wha/economic_conditiond/html. Accessed February 1, 2003

21. Frank M, Reed G. *Denial of Food and Medicine: The Impact of the US Embargo on Health and Nutrition in Cuba.* Washington, DC: American Association for World Health; 1997

22. Garfield R, Santana S. The impact of the economic crisis and the US embargo on health in Cuba. *Am J Public Health.* 1997;87:15–20

23. National Center for Health Statistics. Infant mortality statistics from the 2000 period linked birth/infant death data set. *Natl Vital Stat Rep.* 2002;50. Available at: http://www.cdc.gov/nchc/releases/02facts/ infmort.htm. Accessed February 1, 2003

24. Centers for Disease Control and Prevention. Births, marriages, divorces, and deaths: provisional data for 2001. *Natl Vital Stat Rep.* 2002;50:14

25. Cuban Ministry of Public Health. *Infant Mortality by Provinces: 1975–2001.* Available at: http://www.sld.cu/anuario/anu01/CMT15.htm. Accessed February 1, 2003

26. De la Osa J, Reed G. Cuba registers 6.4 infant mortality: lowest ever. *MEDICC Rev.* 2000;2. Available at: http://www.medicc.org/ Medicc%20Reviews/1999/autum/html/health_news_from_cuba.html. Accessed February 1, 2003

27. National Center for Health Statistics. US infant mortality rate. *Natl Vital Stat Rep.* 2002;50

28. Cuban Ministry of Public Health. *Maternal Mortality by Provinces: 1999–2001.* Available at: http://www.sld.cu/anuario/an01/materna.htm. Accessed February 1, 2003

29. Alternative Medicine Foundation. *Herbmed.* Available at: http://www.amfoundation.org/herbmed.html. Accessed February 1, 2003

30. The Garden Web Plant Database 2000. Available at: http://www.garden web.com/plants/. Accessed February 1, 2003

31. Garcia MM. Saber y Hacer Sobre Plantas Medicinales. Habana, Cuba: 10 de Mayo de 1995

32. GardenInfo. Available at: http://www.gardeninfo.com. Accessed February 1, 2003

33. The Garden Web Plant Database. Available at: http://www.gardenweb.com/plants. Accessed February 1, 2003

34. Growit. Available at: http://www.growit.com. Accessed February 1, 2003

35. Macore Labels. Available at: http://www.macore.com. Accessed February 1, 2003

36. Healthy People 2010. *A Systematic Approach to Health Improvement.* Available at: http://www.healthypeople.gov. Accessed February 1, 2003

37. Arialdi MM, Arias E, Kochanek KD, Murphy SL, Smith BL. Deaths: final data 2000. *Natl Vital Stat Rep.* 2002;50. Available at: http://www.cdc.gov/nchs/fastats/hisfacts.htm. Accessed February 1, 2003

38. Adams DL, ed. *Health Issues for Women of Color.* London, UK: Sage Publications; 1995

39. Rodríguez I, Garcia A, Fernandez I, Lago P, Rodriguez A, Concepcion A. Possible factors associated with epidemic neuropathy in Cuba. *Revista Cubana Med Tropical.* 1998;50:55–60. Available at: http://www.medicc.org/Medicc%20Review/1999/spring/html. Accessed February 1, 2003

40. Hedges TR, Hirano M, Tucker K, Caballero B. Epidemic optic and peripheral neuropathy in Cuba: a unique geopolitical public health problem. *Survey Ophthalmol.* 1997;41:341–353.

41. Ackerman LK. Health problems of refugees. *J Am Board Fam Pract.* 1997;10:337–348

42. Flaskerud JH, Kim S. Health problems of Asian and Latino immigrants. *Nurs Clin North Am.* 1999;34:359–380

43. Juarbe TC. Access to health care for Hispanic women: a primary health care perspective. *Nurs Outlook.* 1995;43:23–28

44. Derose KP, Baker DW. Limited English proficiency and Latinas' use of physician services. *Med Care Res Rev.* 2000;57:76–91

45. National Center for Health Statistics. *Changing America: Indicators of Social and Economic Well-being by Race and Hispanic Origin, 2000.* Available at: http://www.cdc.gov. Accessed February 1, 2003

46. *Cuban Immigration to the USA: Immigrant Visa Processing.* Available at: http://www.wave.net/upg/immigration/cuban_visa.html. Accessed February 1, 2003

47. Pérez JT, Von Braumuhl J, Valencia J, Marquez M. *Cuba's Family Doctor Programme.* Havana, Cuba: Ministry of Public Health; 1996

48. National Coalition of Hispanic Health and Human Services Organization. Meeting the health promotion needs of Hispanic communities. *Am Health Promotion.* 1995;9:300–311

49. Denman-Vitale S, Murillo EK. Effective promotion of breastfeeding among Latin American women newly immigrated to the United States. *Holistic Nurs Pract.* 1999;13:51–60

50. Lederman R, Miller DS. Adaptation to pregnancy in three different ethnic groups: Latin-American, African-American, and Anglo-American. *Can J Nurs Res.* 1998;30:37–51

51. Whiteford LM, Szelag BJ. Access and utility as reflections of cultural constructions of pregnancy. *Primary Care Update Ob/Gyn.* 2000;7:98–104

52. Spector RE. *Cultural Care: Guidelines to Heritage Assessment and Health Traditions.* 2nd ed. Upper Saddle River, NJ: Prentice Hall Health; 2000

53. Gonzalez R. *Cuban Cuisine: As Mulatto as Its People.* New York, NY: Center for Cuban Studies; 2000. Available at: http://www.cubaupdate.org/art22.htm. Accessed February 1, 2003

54. *Cocina Cubana.* Habana, Cuba: Editorial Científico—Técnica; 1997

55. Hayes K. Feeding their own: Cubans turn to soy as an alternative protein source. In: *Blue Book.* 1995. Available at: http://www.soyatech.com/ Cuba.html. Accessed February 1, 2003

56. Orisha Net. *The Religion in Africa and Cuba: How Different Are They Really?* Available at: http://www.seanet.com/~efunmoyiwa/africa.html. Accessed February 1, 2003

57. Kramer EJ, Ivey SL, Ying YW, eds. *Immigrant Women's Health: Problems and Solutions.* San Francisco, CA: Jossey-Bass Publications; 1999

58. Dorticos-Balea A. Reproductive behavior of couples at risk for sickle cell disease in Cuba: a follow-up study. *Prenat Diagn.* 1997;17:737–742

59. Loria CM, Bush TL, Carroll MD, et al. Macronutrient intakes among adult Hispanics: a comparison of Mexican Americans, Cuban Americans, and mainland Puerto Ricans. *Am J Public Health.* 1995;85:684–689

60. Black SA, Markides KS. Acculturation and alcohol consumption in Puerto Rican, Cuban-American, and Mexican-American Women in the United States. *Am J Public Health.* 1993;83:890–893

61. Hernandez BH, Boza AV, Leon EC, Pineda AB. Sexually transmitted diseases in pregnancy. *Rev Cubana Obstet Ginecol.* 1998;24:28–33. Available at: http://www.medicc.org/Medic%20Review/1999/ summer/html/pregnancy.html. Accessed February 1, 2003

62. Reed G, ed. AIDS and a Cuban vaccine update. *MEDICC Rev.* 1999;1:2–5. Available at: http://www.medicc.org/Medicc%20Review/1999/ summer/html/healthnewsfromcuba.html. Accessed February 1, 2003

63. Reed G. AIDS deaths down in Cuba. *MEDICC Rev.* 2001;1. Available at: http://www.medicc.org/medicc%20review/2001/summer-winter/ news.html. Accessed February 1, 2003

64. Matthews TJ, Ventura SJ, Curtin SC, Martin JA. Births of Hispanic origin, 1989-1995. *Monthly Vital Statistics Rep.* 1998;46(6 Suppl):1–28

65. Mendoza JP, Pons OR, Sánchez RB. Male adolescents and contraception. *Rev Cubana Obstet Ginecol.* 1998;24:5–12. Available at: http://www.medicc.org/Medicc%20Review/1999/summer/html/ contraception/html. Accessed February 1, 2003

66. Reed G, ed. Abortion in Cuba: a right and a responsibility. *MEDICC Rev.* 1999;1:5–7. Available at: http://www.medicc.org/Medicc%20Review/ 1999/summer/html/healthnewsfromcuba.html. Accessed February 1, 2003
67. Mendoz JP, Izquiendo AR, Lammers C, Blum, RW. Abortion among adolescents in Cuba. *J Adolesc Health.* 1999;24:59–62

Further Reading

The Jews of Cuba. Available at: http://www.jewishcuba.org. Accessed February 1, 2003

Le Riverend J. *Cuba: Land and People.* 5th ed. Torino, Italy: Mec-Graphic; 1996

Orthosiphon Arestatus Blume. Available at: http://www.pharmacy.cmu.ac.th/pharcog. Accessed February 1, 2003

6
Perinatal Health Care Issues of Hmong Women

Renee B. Neri

Before the Vietnam War, the Hmong were an agrarian people living in small villages in the northern mountains of Laos. Theirs was a simple and primitive culture that didn't even have a written language until 1954.[1] After the American troops left Vietnam in 1975, the Hmong fled to refugee camps in Thailand to escape communist oppression. In the late 1970s they began moving to the United States. Initially they lived scattered in many states. Subsequently families were reunited, and they put down roots in the farming communities of California, Minnesota, Michigan, and Wisconsin.

The Hmong have a strong belief in the existence of a soul, reincarnation, and an afterlife, when their souls will be reunited with those of their ancestors. Elaborate funerals are required or the soul of the dead person may remain in limbo and will be unable to find its ancestors; chanting and playing a reed pipe are used to lead the soul to heaven. Although the traditional religion is a mixture of ancestor worship and animism, some Hmong became Christian in the resettlement camps.[2]

Health and Illness

The Hmong believe that illness occurs when an object has violated the integrity of the body, the spirit has been possessed, the soul lost, or a taboo breached. When they are ill, they turn to the native healers (shaman), who have successfully diagnosed and treated their illnesses for centuries by using herbs, prayers, and other native rituals and remedies.[3]

The Hmong will seek out the services of a Western provider when the native healer has not been able to cure them. However, they find the language barrier as well as the Western provider's lack of understanding about their health beliefs to be significant impediments to care. Moreover, the Hmong have no frame of reference for Western medicine's biomedical framework. For the Hmong, there is no germ theory; thus they are not likely to comply with medical orders that do not agree with their religious or cultural beliefs.[2]

In their native country, members of a Hmong family usually defer decision making to a family elder or the man of the family. This may cause conflicts when they immigrate to the United States and the women try to emulate their American counterparts in controlling their own destinies.[4]

Pregnancy/Prenatal Care

Hmong women view pregnancy as a normal event in life. They do not understand the need for regular prenatal care and are likely to have their first prenatal visit well after the first trimester. An appointment system is not used in their country. Therefore, it is common for them to arrive for care when it fits into their work schedule and family responsibilities.

Every effort should be made to see that the providers and interpreters who care for these women are female. Information about their bodies and the area between the waist and the knees is considered very private.

Hmong women do not readily accept routine prenatal testing. They believe that if blood is taken from the body, it will not be regenerated and they will become very weak as a result. They also feel betrayed by tests that eventually identify problems with which they must then deal.

Although Hmong women do not have any dietary restrictions during pregnancy, they rarely consume dairy products and may be lactose intolerant. They classify foods as hot or cold and sweet or sour[2] and tend to crave the latter. Public assistance vouchers provided by the

Special Supplemental Nutrition Program for Women, Infants, and Children (WIC) should be modified to allow for the purchase of nutritious dairy substitutes that they will eat.

There are many taboos in the Hmong culture. For example, it is commonly believed that if a pregnant woman raises her hands above her head, the baby will not be able to breathe.[1] In addition, the women often wear a string around their waist or wrist to keep the soul in the body; it should not be removed. The Hmong also have a great fear that the soul will leave the body if the integrity of the skin is broken; this is compounded by a fear that general anesthesia will produce memory loss.[4] Thus it is important that such invasive procedures as amniocentesis, episiotomy, cesarean delivery, and circumcision be discussed early in the prenatal period.[1,2] Because family elders are usually involved in major decision making, it may be helpful for the health care provider to participate in a family meeting to ensure informed consent prior to any surgery.[4]

Babies conceived out of wedlock bring shame to the woman and her family; thus in their native country, unmarried pregnant girls were sent to an "old woman" or native healer to get rid of the baby.[1] There is no cultural barrier to terminating a pregnancy because a baby is not believed to exist until the third day after birth when it is named. Consequently, babies lost to miscarriage, stillbirth, or neonatal death may not be acknowledged when a prenatal history is taken.

Labor and Delivery

Most often the Hmong live in large family groups, and in their native country, birth takes place at home. Consequently, they are very afraid when they are alone.[2] In the United States, every effort should be made to see that a Hmong woman is not left alone during labor. If the father is not available, an elder female family member may take his place.

In the Hmong culture, it is believed that pain should be endured. As a result, they will not expect to receive medication to alleviate pain during labor. Most often Hmong women are very stoic, making it difficult to assess the intensity of their contractions without using a monitor or manual palpation. Squatting or sitting tend to be the preferred positions during labor.

Postpartum and Newborn Care

In their native country, Hmong women were confined to bed for 40 days after delivery, staying near a fire to keep warm.[5] In America, most Hmong women have dispensed with the tradition of postpartum confinement because they must resume caring for their families as soon as possible.

During the postpartum period, the husband generally prepares meals. Warm chicken soup is prepared for the Hmong mother soon after delivery. During the first month, her diet consists primarily of chicken, pork, some fish, rice, and eggs, while cold beverages, fruits, and vegetables are usually avoided.[1]

It is widely believed that wearing shoes around a woman who is lactating will dry up her milk[5]; thus shoes should be removed before entering the home of a breastfeeding mother. In the United States, bottle-feeding is opted for more often than breastfeeding because women must return to the workplace as soon as possible. In addition, they tend to view bottle-feeding as more American.[2]

Admiring a Hmong newborn should be avoided. The parents may fear that the admirer wishes to steal the baby's soul. On the third day of life, Hmong babies have a "soul calling" ceremony during which they are given a name. At this time, a small necklace is placed around the baby's neck to keep the soul in the body. This name will be retained for life unless the baby becomes ill and the native healer feels that it may be due to the baby's dislike for his or her name. If this happens, another "soul calling" ceremony is held and a new name is given.[5]

Family Planning

In previous generations, childbearing among Hmong women began at an early age and continued through menopause[3]; hence their fertility rate was high. However, because women exclusively breastfed their babies, pregnancies were naturally spaced from 19 to 22 months apart. Today Hmong women tend to bottle-feed; thus birth control has become a concern as more and more desire to limit the size of their families.

Tubal ligation may be rejected because women fear that their husbands will lose regard for them if they are infertile and that surgery will leave them in a weakened state.[4] Many women are not compliant in taking oral contraceptives[2] or using a diaphragm. Men clearly reject the use of condoms. While the best options for birth control may be the intrauterine device (IUD) and contraceptive implants or injectibles, the persistent bleeding associated with these methods may become a problem.

Death/Burial Rites

In their native land, the Hmong bury the placenta, allowing it to be reclaimed by its owner after death for the journey to join the ancestors in heaven. The placenta of a female child is buried near the mother's bed while the placenta of a male child is buried near the central post of the home. Remarkably, Hmong women have become comfortable with having the placenta "buried" at the hospital.[5]

When a death has occurred, it is very important that there be an elaborate funeral; otherwise, the soul of the dead person may get stuck in limbo and not be able to join his ancestors in heaven. If this happens, the deceased will not be able to be reincarnated into another life. During the funeral service, there will be chanting, and a reed pipe is played to help lead the soul safely to heaven.

Perinatal Health Care Issues of Hmong Women: Key Highlights

Characteristics

- In Vietnam, there is no appointment system; thus in the United States, women may arrive early, late, or not at all for scheduled appointments.
- Health care providers and interpreters should be female.
- Prolonged eye contact may make the patient feel ill at ease.
- Women may not be compliant if medical instructions do not agree with cultural or religious beliefs.
- Traditionally, Hmong religion is a mixture of ancestor worship and animism.
- Some Hmong became Christian in the resettlement camps and believe in the existence of a soul.

Prenatal Care

- Pregnancy is viewed as a normal event.
- Routine prenatal care is a foreign concept.
- Pregnant women should be screened for parasites, tuberculosis, hepatitis B virus, and certain hereditary blood disorders.
- Miscarriages and babies who live less than 3 days may not be acknowledged in the history of previous pregnancies.
- The area of the body between the waist and the knees is considered private and should not be exposed unnecessarily.

Prenatal Testing

- There tends to be a lack of understanding regarding the need for routine prenatal testing.
- Invasive procedures, such as pelvic examinations and ultrasounds, tend to be feared.
- It is commonly believed that blood does not regenerate; thus blood work should be kept to a minimum.

Pregnancy Diet
- No dietary restrictions are observed.
- Foods tend to be classified as hot or cold or sweet or sour.
- Cravings for sweet or sour foods are common.
- Dairy products are rarely consumed; thus WIC vouchers may need to be modified accordingly.

Pregnancy-Related Beliefs/Taboos
- Wearing a string around the waist or wrist may protect the soul from leaving the body.
- Raising one's hand above the head during pregnancy may prevent the baby from breathing.
- Blood samples taken will not regenerate and the person will become very weak.
- The soul will leave the body through any break in the integrity of the skin; thus common obstetric procedures such as amniocentesis, episiotomy, and cesarean birth are feared.
- General anesthesia can produce memory loss.
- Admiring a Hmong newborn may be interpreted as a desire to steal the baby's soul.
- Wearing shoes around a lactating woman can cause the milk to dry up.

Labor and Delivery
- In the United States, the Hmong husband is usually the labor partner.
- Being alone at any time is very frightening to the Hmong woman.
- Squatting or sitting are the preferred positions during labor.
- Pain is to be endured, not alleviated; thus Hmong women may appear stoic during labor.
- In their native country, Hmong women give birth at home; in the United States, they may choose to deliver at home if the hospital is not sensitive to their cultural and religious beliefs.

Postpartum Care
- In their native country, Hmong women are confined to bed for 40 days after giving birth.
- In the United States, new mothers are expected to return to normal responsibilities as soon as possible.

Postpartum Diet
- The Hmong husband generally prepares meals during the early postpartum period.
- The new mother is given warm chicken soup soon after delivery.
- Chicken, pork, fish, rice, and eggs are consumed during the first month after birth; cold beverages, fruits, and vegetables are to be avoided.

Neonatal Care
- On the third day of life, a Hmong baby is given a name in a "soul calling" ceremony.
- A small necklace is placed around the baby's neck to keep the soul in the body.
- Circumcision is generally not done due to the fear that the soul will leave the body through the break in the baby's foreskin.

Breastfeeding/Breast Care
- Breasts are viewed as organs of nutrition with no sexual connotation.
- Women breastfeed almost exclusively in their native country; in the United States, many Hmong women bottle-feed so that they can return to work quickly, and they think it is more American.

Family Planning
- Hmong women have a high fertility rate as a result of beginning childbearing at an early age and ending childbearing at an advanced age.
- In their native country, women exclusively breastfed, which helped to space pregnancies.

- Tubal ligations are not well accepted because women fear that their husbands will find them undesirable if they are infertile; there is also fear that the surgery will make them weak.
- Hmong women may be unreliable in taking oral contraceptives or using a diaphragm.
- Most Hmong men refuse to use condoms.
- IUDs and contraceptive implants or injectibles may be good options.

Family Involvement
- The husband, his mother, and the women elders usually provide support.

Pregnancy Termination/Miscarriage
- Out-of-wedlock pregnancies bring shame and are generally terminated by a native healer.
- There is no cultural barrier to terminating pregnancy because a baby is not believed to exist until the third day after birth when it is named.

Death/Burial Rites
- An elaborate funeral must be held or the soul of the dead person may remain in limbo and be unable to find its ancestors; chanting and playing a reed pipe helps lead the soul to heaven.
- The Hmong strongly believe in an afterlife and reincarnation.

References

1. Faller HS. Perinatal needs of immigrant Hmong women: surveys of women and health care providers. *Public Health Rep.* 1985;100:25–28
2. Muecke MA. Caring for southeast Asian refugee patients in the USA. *Am J Public Health.* 1983;73:431–438
3. Mattson S, Lew I. Culturally sensitive prenatal care for southeast Asians. *J Obstet Gynecol Neonatal Nurs.* 1991;21:48–54
4. Bliatout BT. Hmong attitude towards surgery: how it affects patient prognosis. *Migration World.* 1985;XVI:25–28
5. Lee GL. Cultural identity in post-modern society: reflection of what is Hmong? *Hmong Studies J.* 1996;1–8

7

Perinatal Health Care Issues
of Jamaican Women

Sandra K. Cesario and Deborah Campbell

Jamaica, the third largest island in the Caribbean, is slightly smaller than the state of Connecticut. Located between Cuba and Hispaniola in the Caribbean Sea, its population is currently 2.6 million, with an annual population growth rate of 0.9%, nearly one third of whom are younger than 15 years.[1] There are 2 main urban centers on the island: Kingston on the southeast coast and Montego Bay on the northwest coast. These are home to approximately 55% of the island's residents.[2,3]

Jamaicans come from diverse backgrounds that all have contributed to cultural, educational, and socioeconomic heterogeneity. Theirs is an amalgam of different cultures that emanate from around the world—a blend of old and new. The Caribbean and, more specifically, the Jamaican way of life melds European and African influences, Asian and Middle Eastern components, and new traditions that cannot be traced directly to any other origin than that of the Caribbean.

Most Jamaicans are of mixed race. Today the ethnic composition of Jamaica is 90.4% African descent, 1.3% East Indian, 0.2% white, 7.3% mixed, and 0.6% other, including Chinese.[4-6] The genesis of this racial blending dates back to colonial times when the Spanish and other Europeans brought African slaves to the island. In time Chinese and East Indian workers were also brought to Jamaica.

In 2000 28.4 million foreign-born individuals resided in the United States, representing 10.4% of the total population. Of these, Caribbean immigrants numbered approximately one half million (9.9%),[7] with

59% settling in the northeastern regions of the United States and 31% residing in the south.[8] During the 20th century increasing numbers of Caribbeans fled to North America and Europe because of the economic depression in their homelands. In Jamaica, for example, the high annual inflation and unemployment rates (14.8%) in conjunction with a low per capita income (approximately $3,400 US per person per year), resulted in poverty for nearly one third of the population.[9]

The high rate of Caribbean emigration has resulted in as many Jamaicans residing in the United States, Canada, and the United Kingdom combined as remain on the island.[9] At present the largest concentration of Jamaicans is in New York, New Jersey, and Connecticut.[6] Fifty percent of those employed are women. Among Jamaican residents in the United States are a considerable number of undocumented aliens. These individuals are typically less skilled and tend to be employed in lower paying or more hazardous jobs. Despite this fact, Jamaican immigrants have been more successful economically in terms of income and employment opportunities than black immigrants from other countries.[10] Many Jamaicans travel freely between the United States and Jamaica, earning income that provides financial support for their families at home.

Among the major immigrant groups in the United States, Jamaicans are the only people for whom English is the official primary language. Yet, their ability to speak and understand English depends on education, socioeconomic status, and geographic location of residence. For many, Patois, or Creole, a musical dialect with a uniquely Jamaican rhythm and cadence, is the commonly spoken language among Jamaicans and is spoken in rural and urban communities. Patois is a fusion of English and African languages and reflects the countries from which African slaves were brought to Jamaica in the 15th and 16th centuries.

Formal education in Jamaica is categorized according to 4 levels: pre-primary (early childhood), primary (ages 6–12), secondary (ages

12–17, includes technical and vocational programs), and tertiary (college and university). Education is compulsory through secondary school. The literacy rate, defined as being older than 15 years and having ever attended school, is higher for women (89.1%) than for men (80.8%)[11]; however, many more Jamaicans are functionally illiterate. Although more than 90% of children finish primary school, only about 60% of those eligible children enter secondary school.[9] This is due in large part to the need for older children, especially in rural communities, to enter the workforce to help support their families. While females outnumber males at the secondary school level, more men attend college and university.

Most Jamaicans (55%) are Protestant and either belong to the Church of God, Baptist, Seventh-Day Adventist, Anglican, or Pentecostal religions Four percent are Roman Catholic, and 35% practice other faiths or spiritual cults. Religious practices tend to be ecumenical and often include celebrations of Hindu, Muslim, and Jewish rites. Religion plays an important role in Jamaican society, especially for women and children,[9] and greatly influences the educational system and the expectations of social behavior.[6] Early religious training is at the core of the society's moral code, dictating how people treat each other. Church attendance serves multiple purposes for Jamaicans, strengthening kinships and extended family bonds while creating community alliances that provide for the social, educational, emotional, and financial support needs of its members. Understanding and addressing the spiritual needs of an individual is an important facet of providing holistic care.

In the 1920s the politico-religious Rastafarians, a black self-empowerment movement, arose among the poorest Jamaicans who attributed their extreme poverty and cultural deterioration to white imperialism. These individuals ascribed to the teachings of Ethiopia's Emperor Haile Salassie I. Rastafarians took Salassie's given name, Ras Tafari (Makonnen), in the belief that his was the emissary (embodiment) of God and referred to him as Jah.[12] This religion recognizes the laws set forth in the Old Testament of the Bible, including certain dietary restrictions. Rastafarians wear their hair in dreadlocks and may cover their heads with large distinctive caps or head wraps.[13]

Jamaicans are a very social people and are traditional in their interactions with others. They may greet one another with a simple nod or bow, handshake, hug, or kiss; such gestures are an important acknowledgment, formally and informally, demonstrating respect for the individual. When introduced, a handshake is typically followed by a "Good morning," "Good afternoon," or "Good evening." When meeting an acquaintance or someone new, introductions are formal, requiring use of "Mr," "Mrs/Miss," or the person's professional title. Children also are respectful in their interactions, referring to adults as "Mr" or "Mrs," unless a person is a close family friend, who is then addressed as "Aunt" or "Uncle."

Contemporary Jamaicans possess strong attributes of confidence, persistence, resilience, resistance, and independence.[5] They are autonomous thinkers who feel it important to be self-reliant and make their own decisions. Some Jamaicans seem confrontational, objecting to others telling them what they should do, that a problem cannot be solved, that a particular goal is not achievable. Their personal pride may impede their relationships with health care professionals and service providers. This may be manifested in different ways. Some may be embarrassed to accept public assistance. Others may reject authority when they perceive that their beliefs are being disregarded or when a caregiver or authority figure is perceived to be condescending. Jamaicans' behavior, although clearly the result of their life's struggle, is often interpreted by others unfamiliar with the culture as aggressive, pushy, and defiant, contributing to misunderstanding and miscommunication.

Family relationships vary among Jamaicans, reflecting the vestiges of slavery and colonialism. Extended families are the norm in

Jamaica,[6] with grandparents residing in the home of one of their children, and children remaining in their parents' home into adulthood. Household size varies, but averages 3.6 people per family. Women head approximately 44% of all households[14] and have 2 to 3 children on average. Women in rural communities tend to have more children than those living in urban communities. Kinship bonds are characteristically strong. Aunts and uncles are considered close family members and often are viewed as surrogate parents. They play a significant role in family life and childrearing, often providing emotional and financial support. Jamaicans have a strong sense of community and support for one another.

The family structure of upper- and middle-class Jamaicans more commonly embodies European standards and values, including formal marriages. Cohabitation is viewed with shame and moral guilt and is deemed an unacceptable lifestyle because it does not legitimize any offspring and, thus, lowers the family's social status. Furthermore, the choice of a marriage partner requires careful consideration of the potential spouse's socioeconomic, educational, and cultural background. Occupation, financial independence, skin color, and the family's status within the community are also important considerations.

The residual effects of slavery on family structure and sexual behavior remain evident among poor and lower-class Jamaicans.[6] Traditional island families in lower socioeconomic groups tend to be larger than those in the middle or upper classes.[4,11] There is no cultural stigma attached to lower-income women having several children with different men known as "baby fathers." Likewise, the male partners refer to these women as "baby mothers" instead of wives or girlfriends. Cohabitation is very common, with members of the community recognizing the couple as husband and wife.

An unusual facet of Jamaican life is the occurrence of "visiting unions." These are additional intimate relationships outside the legal marriage or primary cohabitation partnership. It is reported that between 20% to 35% of Jamaican men are involved in these types of relationships.[15] Many Jamaican men will have more than one partner at a time, and children frequently result from these extra unions. The existence of visiting unions and more than one family is not unique to the lower classes and may be seen among professional men as well. Visiting unions often develop for men who must travel to different parts of the island or outside of the country for employment purposes.

An important factor in the deterioration of the traditional family structure is the need for migration outside of Jamaica, typically for employment purposes. Although many individuals emigrate with the intention of reuniting with their children, often this fails to happen. Children remain behind in Jamaica to be raised by relatives, friends, or neighbors. The absent parents will send money and goods back to their children and family, but may not be able to reunite with their children for many years, if at all. Among emigrants, it is not uncommon to have 2 or more families living together for financial and social support.

Because fathers may be away from home for long periods or minimally involved, childrearing and decision making are considered to be the woman's domain. It is generally the woman's responsibility to manage the finances, as well as to discipline and educate the children. The female caregiver in the family is often held responsible for a child's misbehavior or poor performance. Independent and strong-willed, Jamaican women model these qualities for their daughters and younger women in their family.

Within traditional Caribbean culture, the concept of manhood is based almost exclusively on 3 elements: sexuality or sexual identity, a man's primary role as a provider to his family, and scriptural authority for man as the family's head.[15–18] Unfortunately, Jamaican boys and young men receive mixed messages about what it means to be a man. Boys are encouraged by their peers and male family members to become sexually active at a young age. Losing one's virginity, having multiple partners, and fathering or "getting" a child are considered important signs of manhood.[18,19] This is distinguished from "having" children, which implies responsibility for the maintenance and care of that child.[19] The ability to provide for their children is often of little consequence to younger men. This commonly leads to low expectations for fathers with regard to raising their children beyond the provision of financial support. In addition, unemployment and underemployment have created a significant barrier to men fulfilling their perceived role as provider. On the other hand, Jamaican men frequently contribute more than they are given credit for. Men are far more involved in positively contributing to family life than stereotypes often suggest.[16] Although men rarely depict their role as nurturers for their children, they do describe their daily involvement in providing physical care for, playing with, and disciplining their children as well as other domestic tasks. For fathers who reside with their children, there tends to be common acceptance of financial responsibility, but variations in their understanding about the social and psychological components of fathering.[16] Among younger men with families, attitudes are changing and their involvement in daily family life seems to be increasing.

Distrust and disillusionment frequently characterize the female-male relationship and may be attributable to each gender's differing perceptions of fidelity, men's ultimate power and authority, expectations of men as the primary family provider, the division of domestic tasks across traditional gender lines, and domestic violence.[17] Although violence against women is widespread, with 9% of women reporting being victims of physical abuse,[3] many women are reluctant to acknowledge or report abusive behavior. In Jamaica, despite the passage of a Domestic Violence Act in 1995, there is little public awareness or enforcement of the law.[3] Nearly 45% of the murders on the island are reported to be the result of domestic violence. Among adolescent females aged 15 to 19 years, 26% report having experienced forced sexual intercourse.[3] As is true in the United States, many of these women are dependent on their abusive partners for financial support, have few options, and are fearful and embarrassed by their situation.

Health and Illness

The maternal mortality rate in 2000 was reported to be 110 deaths per 100,000 live births.[20] Infant mortality rates in Jamaica have shown marked improvement over the last 10 years, declining from 29.8 deaths per 1,000 live births in 1990 to an estimated 14.2 deaths per 1,000 live births in 2001.[20] This improvement can be primarily attributed to improved care for preterm infants, infants with congenital defects, and diarrheal conditions. The incidence of low birth weight remains fairly steady at 11%.[21] Over the past 5 years, immunization coverage of children younger than 1 year has increased steadily to almost 90%.[22]

Although standards of health care are reasonably high in Jamaica, hospitals are few and a system of community-based health care clinics predominates. Private health care is available for those who can afford it; however, most health care services are provided for free or at low cost in public facilities. Jamaicans tend to self-medicate and will try various home remedies before seeking medical attention. Routinely, it is the women who assume responsibility for securing health care services for themselves and their families, and, typically, their children's health and resource needs are always put first.

The spiritual use of marijuana (ganja) is an important facet of Rastafarian life for men. Ganja, also known as Indian hemp, is more potent than marijuana from the West and is capable of producing hallucinations. Although the male-dominated rural ganja culture specifically states that women should not routinely smoke ganja, many women do so. In fact, it is estimated that as many as 50% of Jamaican women smoke ganja; for non-Rastafarian women, it is often a clandestine activity. In addition, the medicinal use of ganja in the form of tinctures and teas is often recommended.

Obesity and smoking, especially among women, have dramatically increased the incidence of hypertension and cancer among Jamaicans over the last 20 years. Reportedly, cancer of the breast (the number 1 cause of death), cervix, and stomach kill more than 2,000 Jamaican women each year, many of them at a very young age.[23] In addition, more than one half of the adult women and one quarter of the men are reported to be obese,[24] an alarming trend that may be attributed to the increased consumption of carbohydrates and fast foods that are typically high in salt, sugar, and fat calories. Those who lead more sedentary lifestyles further compound their risk for diabetes, heart disease, and strokes.

The Jamaican diet reflects a fusion of the various ethnic influences that make up the populace. Minerals, including calcium, potassium, magnesium, and phosphorus, are plentiful, as is dietary fiber.[25] Carbohydrates are derived primarily from rice, yams, sweet potatoes, ackee, breadfruit, plantains (green bananas), peas, and pumpkin. Tropical fruits such as bananas, coconuts, mangoes, papayas, pineapples, oranges, and grapefruits are also consumed abundantly. Bammy, or cassava bread, a bland hard dough bread, is another common staple in their diet. Protein sources come from poultry, fresh and salted fish, shellfish, beef, pork, and goat (mutton). Protein portions are typically small, with an average serving size weighing 3 oz.[6] Foods are highly seasoned and spicy. Infusions made from boiled roots, herbal teas, fruit juices, and a variety of alcoholic drinks are common; coffee, cocoa, and tea are consumed freely. Their main meal is typically taken midday. In contrast, Rastafarians eat what is known as an I-tal diet, based on raw, organic foods: vegetables, fruits, nuts, and seeds. Forbidden foods include pork, shellfish, and alcohol, while coffee and salt are discouraged. Some Rastafarians do eat fish, however. See Table 7.1 and Glossary.

Approximately 60% of Jamaican teenagers are sexually experienced; indeed, the mean age for first intercourse is reported to be 14[7] years

Table 7-1
Jamaican Food Preferences

Protein	Dairy	Grains	Vegetables	Fruits	Other
Salt fish*	Goats milk	Bammy*	Yams	Ackee*	Beverages
Stews		Rice	Peas	Green	Coffee
Chicken		Fried	Red beans	bananas	Herbal teas
Curried goat		dumplings	Lettuce	Mangoes	Fruit juices
Jerk*		Bunuelos	Tomatoes	Papayas	Cocoa
Pork		Coo-coo*	Cabbage	Pineapple	Beer
Bistec a la		Yucca	Carrots	Oranges	Rum
criolla*		Bulla*	Pimienta*	Grapefruit	Wine
Marlin		Callaloo*	Aranitas*	Star fruit	
Boudin*		Calabaza*	Breadfruit*	Cherimoya*	Spices
Chorizo		Cassava*	Chili peppers	Guava	Annatto*
Conch			Chayote*	Limes	Arrowroot
Jack*			Malanga*	Mamey	Blaff*
Lobster			Okra	apples	Cassareep*
Shrimp			Onion	Matrimony*	Nutmeg
Crab			Mannish		Stinking
Escoveitch			water*		toe*
fish*					Tamarind*
Run down or					Cilantro
"run dun"*					

*See Glossary.

for girls[3] and 13.4 years for boys.[26] Such early sexual activity has increased their risks for pregnancy, physical or sexual abuse, and sexually transmitted diseases (STDs), including human immunodeficiency virus (HIV) and acquired immunodeficiency syndrome (AIDS). Reportedly, 50% of sexually active teens in 1998 did not use any form of contraception[3]; of these, more than 80% of them had unplanned or unwanted births in 2000.[26] Jamaica's adolescent pregnancy rate is among the highest in the Caribbean, with 40% of Jamaican women having been pregnant at least once before the age of 20 years. Of concern is that some males may coerce their partners into having unprotected sex because of their preference for skin-to-skin contact; this is particularly worrisome because 60% of girls younger than 13 years are estimated to have had their first sexual encounter with men 6 years their senior.[19] Misconceptions that contraception causes infertility, brain damage, infection, and memory loss, or that sex with a virgin can cure an STD, only add to a teen's confusion about reproductive issues.

The number of people with HIV and AIDS continues to increase among Jamaicans.[26] The major route of spread of HIV and AIDS in the Caribbean is heterosexual transmission, primarily affecting the reproductive age group. The risk factors most prevalent among HIV-infected individuals are a history of STDs (39%) and multiple sex partners (32%).[27] Jamaica's highest infection rate occurs among individuals aged 15 to 24 years,[28] with one third of the cases involving women. In 1998 43% of new cases were infected women.[3] Each year 7.5% of HIV-infected women give birth; on average, 1 baby per day is born to an HIV-positive mother on the island. Nevirapine therapy is used in labor to reduce mother-to-infant transmission.

Although STDs are the third leading reason for health center visits among young women in Jamaica, their prevalence has decreased in recent years, with fewer reported cases of chancroid; herpes; ophthalmia neonatorum; and primary, secondary, and tertiary syphilis. The incidences of infections in decreasing order of frequency are gonorrhea (20%), syphilis (7.4%), and herpes (1.7%).[3,27] The Jamaican Ministry of Health has established standards promoting cancer prevention during the reproductive years and has instituted breast and cervical cancer screening at all health centers. In addition, the integration of STD detection and treatment, family planning services, and outreach to fathers-to-be is being encouraged.[3]

Entrenched belief systems play a significant role in Jamaican attitudes about health problems. Illness and disability may be attributed to natural causes, or they may be viewed as an error in medical judgment, caused by germs, or the result of a failed treatment. Many, including some professional and middle-class Jamaicans, view illness and disability as punishment for some transgression or the result of evil spirits (*obeah* or *guzu* [supernatural forces], *duppies,* or ghosts).[3]

Jamaicans generally believe in the power of God to intercede in their lives and mediate between good and evil. There is a dichotomous perspective about God's power and authority: He is punishing, yet forgiving of the sinner. Literal in their interpretation of the Bible, God may be perceived as exacting vengeance on multiple generations. Thus an illness or disability may be viewed as punishment for an evil committed by someone in a previous generation (parent or grandparent). This results in tremendous shame and guilt if a mother herself is blamed for her child's birth defect or illness (ie, failing to go for prenatal care or high-risk care if a problem was suspected). In general, physical illness or disability is accepted more easily than cognitive or mental deficits.

Pregnancy/Prenatal Care

Entry into prenatal care for women in Jamaica generally occurs during the second trimester. A perinatal morbidity and mortality survey[28] indicated that Jamaican women who did not present themselves for prenatal care were more likely to be teenagers, unmarried, in unions of very short duration, smokers, and women without adequate support systems. In addition, women who worked outside the home, had previously uneventful pregnancies, and had short inter-pregnancy intervals were more likely to receive inadequate prenatal care. The tendency for Jamaicans to self-treat, even during pregnancy, makes it essential for the health care provider to be explicit in directions regarding when and for what specific problems the pregnant woman should seek medical attention.

Women of Jamaican descent tend to have a slightly higher incidence of diabetes, anemia, and sickle cell anemia compared with the general US population. According to World Health Organization criteria, Jamaican women 15 years and older have a diabetes prevalence rate of 17.9%.[29] Thus screening for altered glucose tolerance during pregnancy is an important aspect of prenatal care for this population. Iron deficiency anemia, occurring in 7.6% of adolescent Jamaican females, necessitates monitoring of hemoglobin and hematocrit during pregnancy.[30] All pregnant Jamaicans should also be tested for sickle hemoglobin, the abnormal hemoglobin that results in sickle trait or sickle cell anemia. It is noteworthy that Jamaica is home to The Jamaican Sickle Cell Unit, an accredited clinic of the University Hospital of the West Indies, that has focused on studies of the natural history of sickle cell disease to determine some of the factors influencing the severity of the disease.

Rubella is endemic in many Caribbean countries, despite governmental initiatives to eradicate the disease. In 1998 more than 20,000 infants were born with congenital rubella syndrome in Latin American and Caribbean countries.[31] Therefore, determination of rubella status in Jamaican women is essential and should be accompanied by necessary health care instructions to avoid contracting the disease during pregnancy. Post-delivery immunization is recommended if the client is not immune to rubella.

Caribbean food beliefs related to pregnancy are attributed to specific outcomes. For example, the consumption of milk, eggs, tomatoes, and green vegetables is believed to result in a baby that is too large to deliver vaginally. It is also believed that drinking too much liquid will drown the baby. Many Jamaican women expect to experience cravings during their pregnancies and fear that the failure to satisfy the food craving may result in a poor pregnancy outcome. Satisfying the craving seems to be more important than the specific food items themselves. Jamaican women need culturally appropriate counseling about good prenatal nutrition, stressing the need for a diet that is rich in vitamins and minerals, particularly iron.[6]

Chronic stress and depression may be significant issues for pregnant and parenting Jamaican women residing in the United States, particularly if they are separated from all or part of their families.

143

The inability to reunite with their loved ones, concerns related to their children in Jamaica, or perinatal problems arising with a current pregnancy or birth can intensify these feelings. It is therefore important to assess the psychosocial factors that may impede a woman's compliance with care, contribute to deteriorating mental health for the pregnant and/or parenting Jamaican woman, and/or be an impetus to an adverse perinatal outcome for her fetus.

Ganja is often used medicinally during pregnancy. It may be smoked in the first trimester to relieve nausea, vomiting, and fatigue and during the labor process to alleviate the physical and psychological discomfort associated with childbirth, a practice that is discouraged in Jamaica. Prenatal care providers as well as members of the community warn pregnant women about the potential dangers to the fetus; however, there is no conclusive research that the use of marijuana is harmful during the birthing process, and this practice continues in Jamaica, especially in rural areas of the island.[32] Rastafarian women believe that ganja inherently offers medical and spiritual benefits, enhances health and strength, and improves academic performance. Non-Rasta women feel that ganja alleviates the psychological and physical pains associated with being poor and pregnant. In the context of this belief, quitting smoking during pregnancy may not seem logical to the Jamaican woman.[33]

Labor and Delivery

The same warmth, care, and good humor that are apparent in everyday Jamaican life and culture characterize the birth experience. Jamaican women are demonstrative and verbal in response to pain and the childbirth process. Traditionally, other women attend to the labor needs of the parturient, and the labor support network may be very large.[34] Visitation policies and physical facilities of labor and delivery units should, thus, consider the need to accommodate the desire for many individuals to attend the birth. A qualitative study conducted in the United Kingdom revealed that Afro-Caribbean women did not want to be subjected to high-tech procedures, such as fetal monitoring, and viewed childbirth as a natural body function.[35]

Postpartum and Newborn Care

Traditional postpartum care in most Jamaican hospitals is provided in wards of 6 or more women who have recently given birth. There, experienced mothers offer advice and guidance to first-time mothers about infant care, breastfeeding, and recovery from childbirth; all are there for each other in an unspoken sisterhood. Young mothers learn how to breastfeed, diaper, wrap, hold, and soothe their babies by following the example of the more experienced Jamaican mothers. The preference for privacy in the United States contrasts with the Jamaican love for community and may cause distress or a feeling of further isolation for newly immigrated Jamaican mothers.[36]

Postpartum depression was generally uncommon among earlier generations of Jamaican women. Today, however, the changing social structure and increasing poverty in Jamaica seem to have given impetus to a higher rate of postpartum illnesses. It has been suggested that postpartal dysfunctions are a result of inadequate (1) social structuring of postpartum events, (2) social recognition of a role transition for the new mother, (3) meaningful assistance to the new mother, (4) information regarding child care and self-care, and (5) cultural rituals that integrate motherhood into the social order.[37] These phenomena are now thought to affect modern Jamaican women, at home and abroad.

Although breastfeeding promotion has been a national priority in Jamaica since the mid-1970s, the practice is declining within the population.[38] Only 51% of infants seen at postnatal clinics islandwide were reported to be fully breastfed.[22] Infants are usually weaned from the breast by 6 weeks of age with a porridge made from cornmeal, banana, plantain, and/or oats. Beliefs related to infant feeding traditionally center around issues of hot and cold; thus giving a baby a cold bottle or exposing the infant to cold air can result in colic.

On the other hand, breast milk is thought to sour if the mother gets too hot, and sour milk is considered bad for the baby. Caribbean mothers also believe that young children need to be purged to be healthy, and infants and children are given "laxative tonics" for stomachaches. During the purging process, the child is only given teas, thin porridges, or watery soups for nourishment.

Many Jamaicans believe that ghosts or spirits are fond of babies. To protect the child from harm, a Bible opened to one of the Psalms will be placed at the head of the infant's bed.[3] In addition, a black or red string may be tied to the infant's wrist or foot to protect against evil spirits. Accidents and congenital malformations are often attributed to punishment that is deserved. Some parents who give birth to a child with a birth defect may reject that child, while others may overprotect the child with an illness or disability, fostering a sense of vulnerability and dependency by characterizing the child as "sickly."[3] In either event, families grieve intensely over any child's lost potential.

Family Planning

Although public health clinics provide a full range of counseling and contraceptive services in Jamaica, they are not fully used. One study estimates that only 50% to 60% of women use contraception,[3] while another estimates that 18% of married women in the Caribbean have an unmet need for contraception.[39] A barrier to accessing family planning services is the requirement for women to first produce a negative pregnancy test or assert that she is menstruating. Injectable forms of contraceptives are preferred.[6] Women in Jamaica tend to have limited knowledge about emergency contraception. Some may blame a late menses on an unhealthy blockage or an obstruction and take a variety of herbs or other substances (such as the cure-all "washout") to "unblock" menstruation and restore health.[40] Such beliefs and practices provide women with some control over pregnancy, while leaving intact the high value placed on fertility by this culture. To counter the competing socioeconomic and cultural forces in Jamaica that encourage early sexuality and parenthood among adolescents, school-based sexuality education programs have been implemented in grade 7 of public schools and found to be effective in increasing the use of contraception by adolescents.[41]

Sterilization is rare and pregnancy termination is illegal in Jamaica, except to save the life of the mother or protect her physical or mental health.[3] Nevertheless, it is estimated that 1.5% of Jamaican women have had a least one abortion; in fact, complications related to unsafe abortions are one of the leading causes of maternal mortality.[41] As a consequence of inadequate health and family planning programs in their native country, Jamaican women living in the United States may not be familiar with the contraceptive methods or reproductive options available to them or how to access them.

Death/Burial Rites

As with every culture, people of Afro-Caribbean descent have different funeral rites and idiosyncratic beliefs about death and dying. A unifying theme with all cultures, however, is that death and bereavement are distressing times and marked by special ceremonies and expressions of respect paid to the deceased and the deceased's family. Although traditional Jamaican burial practices have evolved over the years, some Jamaicans observe a mourning period called Ni nights (9 nights), during which the bereaved gather to pay their respects, pray, talk, and sing hymns. This offers important support to the family and ensures they are not left alone in their grief. In addition, it is believed to be necessary to ensure the body's safe journey to the next part of life. This ritual is usually held in a veranda or a bamboo and coconut tent next to a house. Fried fish and bread sit on a central table that is left until midnight so that the spirit of the dead may enter and partake of the snack. The ceremony also involves dancing, extensive singing, and 100-proof rum. It ends 9 nights after the death, although additional singing must occur 40 nights later, when the soul is believed to cease roaming the earth and will no longer pester the living. Journey cakes (johnnycakes) are also laid with corpses to provide nourishment as the soul travels to the next world. *Obedah,* or voodoo ceremonies, may take place to help put souls to rest.

The coffin is typically left open for viewing and may be in the home or at the church. The burial ceremony includes family members carrying the coffin to the grave site and taking turns filling the grave with soil.[42] Funerals often feature professional singers and processions. Autopsies are rare. In rural areas, the body may be preserved with ice, weights, and cotton until burial 3 days after the wake.

Based on the strength of their religious convictions, there is a strong belief in the afterlife. Bereavement is considered a private matter and is often not explored because the bereaved are expected to recover quickly and move on with life.[43] Although Jamaicans believe in the sanctity of life, they are somewhat fatalistic. They may believe that no matter what is done, certain conditions, such as breast cancer or having an infant with congenital anomalies, are predestined.[44]

Rastafarians believe that visitation and prayer are very important aspects of support for the sick and dying. Although they do not believe in an afterlife and life is viewed as eternal, passing from one generation to the next, Rastafarians do not have any special ceremonies for the dead. However, burial is their preference following death.

Every Jamaican Woman Is Unique

Provision of perinatal health care for a Jamaican woman is generally interactive and rewarding. The presence of many family members and friends, their animated and demonstrative behaviors, and the lively conversation add to the excitement of the childbirth situation. The diversity of ethnic backgrounds in the Jamaican population makes each birthing experience unique, incorporating a wide variety of beliefs, practices, and religious perspectives into the process. Individualized care is the key to promoting positive birth outcomes. Failure to understand and interpret culturally relevant issues can result in provider and patient frustration and decreased access and quality of care for Jamaican women.

Perinatal Health Care Issues of Jamaican Women: Key Highlights

Demographic/Psychosocial/Spiritual Characteristics

- Jamaican immigrants comprise 9.9% of the foreign-born population in the United States.
- Approximately half a million Jamaicans live in the United States, primarily in the northeast and southern states.
- Patois is the commonly spoken, but unofficial, language.
- High rates of poverty and unemployment necessitate immigration of many Jamaicans to the United States, Canada, and Britain, separating families who may or may not reunite.
- Jamaican women are generally independent and persistent; they tend to be the primary decision makers in the family.
- Separation from their children and the economic impact of poverty may have serious effects contributing to chronic stress, depression, or other mental illnesses.
- Rastafarians have differing practices and beliefs from non-Rastafarian Jamaicans.
- A sense of fatalism underlies some Jamaicans' acceptance of adverse events.
- Due to the prevalence of violence against women in Jamaica, it is important to assess for ongoing intimate partner abuse or the residual effects of prior abuse.
- Early initiation of sexual activity is common among Jamaican women.
- Pregnancy outside of marriage is accepted among lower income women.

Prenatal Care

- Ganja is used by some Jamaican women during pregnancy.
- Depending on the relationship between the couple, Jamaican men may not participate actively in prenatal health care visits or childbirth classes.

- Entry into prenatal care is more common during the second trimester in Jamaica.
- Women whose previous pregnancies were uneventful may not seek health care during subsequent pregnancies.

Prenatal Testing
- Prevalence rates of diabetes and anemia in the Jamaican population are higher than those of the overall US population.
- STDs should be screened for, especially among adolescents.
- A variety of myths and erroneous beliefs increase the adolescent girl's risk for STDs, pregnancy, and abuse.
- Despite decreasing incidence of STDs among Jamaican women, HIV infection continues to increase.
- HIV transmission is predominantly heterosexual or perinatally acquired.
- HIV, sickle cell anemia, and rubella immune status are important risk factors to screen for among pregnant Jamaican women.
- The use of folk remedies, teas and herbs, and marijuana (ganja) should be assessed.
- Psychosocial assessment or screening for depression and other mental health problems is important.

Pregnancy Diet
- The ginger plant, a botanical relative of marjoram and turmeric, is eaten to combat the nausea associated with pregnancy.
- Rastafarian women eat only fresh organic fruits, vegetables, and seeds; they avoid meat, shellfish, salt, alcohol, and empty calorie foods, but may eat fish.

Pregnancy-Related Beliefs and Taboos
- The consumption of milk, eggs, tomatoes, and green vegetables may result in a baby that is too large to deliver vaginally.
- Drinking too much liquid will drown the baby.
- Failure to satisfy a food craving may result in a poor pregnancy outcome.

Labor and Delivery

- Labor needs are typically supported by other women.
- Many people may desire to attend the birth.
- Jamaican women may be demonstrative and verbal in response to pain.
- Pain relief is a priority, and ganja may be used medicinally.
- High-tech procedures are not viewed as desirable.

Postpartum Care

- Rubella immunization may be necessary at the time of postpartum discharge because many Jamaican women are nonimmune.
- Routine Pap smears and breast self-examination are important in light of the increasing incidence of breast and cervical cancers among Jamaican women.
- Postpartum depression is on the rise in this population.
- Traditional postpartal care in Jamaica is a social event, where new mothers learn from each other and exchange stories of life and parenting.

Postpartum Diet

- Other than religious restrictions, no particular rituals are followed.
- Dairy intake is very limited in the Jamaican population.
- Traditional salty, spicy foods may be eaten.

Neonatal Care

- The infant mortality rate in Jamaica has improved dramatically during the last decade, and in 2001 was estimated at 14.2 deaths per 1,000 live births.
- The incidence of low birth weight is 11%.
- The immunization rate is 90% for infants younger than 1 year in Jamaica.
- Jamaican beliefs regarding illness, the birth of a baby with congenital abnormalities, and disability include belief that this occurs as punishment for a past transgression, resulting in tremendous shame and guilt among families.

- Infancy conditions are attributed to the effects of hot and cold.
- Colic can result from cold milk or cold air.
- Breast milk can sour if the mother gets too hot.
- Infants and children need to be "purged" to be healthy.

Breastfeeding and Breast Care
- The rate of breastfeeding is low among Jamaican mothers.
- Those infants breastfed are often weaned by 6 weeks of age.
- The breast cancer rate in Jamaican women is high.

Family Planning
- There are significant knowledge gaps regarding all aspects of women's health and preventive care.
- 18% of married women in the Caribbean have an unmet need for contraception.
- Jamaica has implemented school-based sexuality education in grade 7.

Family Involvement
- The inclusion of the extended family is important to all aspects of family life.
- Female-headed households exceed 50% in parts of the Caribbean.
- Lower income women may have several children with different men known as "baby fathers."

Pregnancy Termination and Miscarriage
- Herbs or other substances (such as the cure-all "washout") are used to "unblock" menstruation and restore health.
- Abortion is one of the leading causes of maternal mortality in Jamaica.

Death and Burial Rites
- Jamaicans are deeply religious; their practices and beliefs are based on their religious and ethnic heritage, but often include aspects of other religions in an ecumenical fashion.

- Jamaicans consider death and mourning a private matter to be attended to by family and friends.
- There is an expectation that grief should be handled quickly and "put to rest" so that the bereaved can return to life's "normal" routine as quickly as possible.
- Extended mourning periods, such as 9-night celebrations, are still practiced.
- Rituals are an important aspect of the grieving process and important in terms of ensuring the deceased's ascension to the afterlife.
- In some communities, obeah, or voodoo ceremonies, may still occur to put the soul to rest.
- Rastafarians do not believe in an afterlife; life is viewed as eternal moving from one generation to the next.

Glossary[45,46]

Ackee: A bright red fruit that grows on an ornamental tree, when ripe it bursts open and reveals 3 large black seeds and a bright yellow flesh. Ackee is a popular breakfast food in Jamaica and resembles scrambled eggs when cooked.

Annatto: A musky-flavored reddish yellow spice, ground from the seeds of a flowering tree and stored in oil.

Aranitas: Fried "spiders" made of julienne strips of green plantain.

Bammy: Cassava bread, a fried dough that is considered a staple food often prepared with fish.

Bistec a la Criolla: Marinated steak, typically rump, round, or sirloin of beef.

Blaff: A broth infused with whole Scotch bonnet peppers and bay rum leaves in which fish are poached.

Boudin: Sausage that may include pigs' blood, thyme, and Scotch bonnet peppers.

Breadfruit: A large, green fruit, usually about 10 in. in diameter, with a pebbly green skin and potatolike flesh that is cooked and served in place of any starchy vegetable, rice, or pasta. It can also be prepared like squash (baked, grilled, fried, boiled, roasted, or stuffed with meat).

Bulla: A ginger sweetcake.

Callaloo: Leafy, spinachlike vegetable.

Calabaza: Large pumpkin used in stews and vegetable dishes.

Cassareep: An important component of Caribbean island stews that is made from grated cassava root and flavored with cinnamon, cloves, and sugar.

Cassava: A tuber also known as manioc and yuca. It is 6 in. to 12 in. in length and 2 in. to 3 in. in diameter and has tough brown skin with a very firm white flesh.

Cherimoya: Pale green fruit with white sweet flesh that has the texture of flan.

Chayote: Small pear-shaped vegetable, light green or cream colored, used as a side dish or in gratins and soufflés. It is also a meat tenderizer.

Coo-coo: The Caribbean equivalent of polenta or grits.

Escoveitch Fish: Pickled fish served with "festival," a deep-fried, sweet cornbread.

Jack: A family of more than 200 different species of colorful saltwater fish.

Jerk: The process of spicing and grilling meats, poultry, and even vegetables, although the most popular is jerk chicken and jerk pork. The process produces foods with a spicy-sweet flavor and a tender texture.

Malanga: A starchy tuber similar to dasheen or taro.

Mamey Apple: A large tropical fruit that yields edible pulp that is tangerine in color and similar in flavor to a peach. It is often made into jam.

Mannish Water: A soup of vegetables and goat meat prepared by boiling the head of a goat in broth.

Matrimony: Orange segments with crushed apples in cream.

Run Down: Fish prepared with coconut milk and spices.

Stinking Toe: A pod that resembles a human toe yielding a sugary powder that can be eaten like candy or made into a flavorful custard or beverage.

Tamarind: A decorative tree that produces brown pods containing a sweet and tangy pulp used in a wide variety of sauces, beverages, and curries. It is also an important ingredient in Jamaican folk medicine.

References

1. Center for Reproductive Law and Policy. *Jamaica Statistics.* Available at: http://www.crlp.org/ww_sbr_jamaica.html. Accessed February 1, 2003
2. Statistical Institute of Jamaica. *Jamaican Statistics, 2001.* Available at: http://www.statinja.com/stats.html. Accessed February 1, 2003
3. The Center for Reproductive Law and Policy. *Women of the World: Jamaica. Laws and Policies Affecting Their Reproductive Lives: Latin America and the Caribbean, Progress Report 2000.* New York, NY: The Center for Reproductive Law and Policy; 2001
4. *Culturgram 2000. Jamaica.* Provo, UT: Brigham Young University; 1999
5. US Central Intelligence Agency. Jamaica. In: *The World Factbook.* Washington, DC: US Central Intelligence Agency; 2003. Available at http://www.cia.gov/cia/publications/factbook/geos/jm.html. Accessed July 21, 2003
6. Miller D. *An Introduction to Jamaican Culture for Rehabilitation Providers.* Buffalo, NY: The Center for International Rehabilitation Research and Information Exchange, State University of New York at Buffalo; 2002
7. Lollock L. *The Foreign-Born Population in the United States. Current Population Reports.* Washington, DC: US Census Bureau; 2000
8. US Immigration and Naturalization Service. *Immigration Fact Sheet 1996.* Washington, DC: Bureau of the Census; 2001

9. *Life, People, Religion, Culture and Lifestyle in Jamaica.* Available at: http://www.scherp.com/culture.htm. Accessed February 1, 2003

10. Grosfogue R. *Afro-Carib Migrations to the United States.* Available at: http://www.africana.com/Articles/tt_426.htm. Accessed February 1, 2003

11. US Central Intelligence Agency. Jamaica—government, history, population, geography, and maps. In: *World Factbook.* Washington, DC: US Central Intelligence Agency. Available at: http://www.worldrover.com/vital/jamaica.html. Accessed February 1, 2003

12. Napti P. *Jamaicans of Ethiopian Origin and the Rastafarian Faith.* Available at: http://web.syr.edu/~affellem/napti.html. Accessed February 1, 2003

13. *Rastafarian Culture and Religion.* Available at: http://il.essortment.com/rastafraincult_reci.htm. Accessed February 1, 2003

14. Lewis M. *Problems in Women's Health and Welfare Infrastructure: Experience From Jamaica.* Jamaica: Planning and Evaluation Unit, Ministry of Health; 2001

15. Stewart M. The changing role of fathers. Presented at: 4th Caribbean Early Childhood Development Conference; July 24, 2002; Georgetown, Guyana

16. Brown J. Gender relations and conflicts in fathering. In: *Coordinator's Notebook.* No. 16, 1995. The Consultative Group on ECCD. Washington, DC: World Book, 1999

17. Brown J, Chevannes B. Redefining fatherhood: a report from the Caribbean. *Early Child Matters.* 2001;97

18. *Jamaica: Mixed Messages on Sexuality.* Available at: http://www.arches.uga.edu/~dionnepages/issue2/One_Love.html. Accessed February 1, 2003

19. Lobban M. Caribbean health: STDs running wild among the region's young. *InterPress News Service.* March 18, 1996. Available at: http://www.aegis.com/news/ips/1996/IP960303.html. Accessed February 1, 2003

20. US Central Intelligence Agency. *The World Fact Book.* Washington, DC: US Central Intelligence Agency; 2001. Available at: http://www.bartleyby.com/151/. Accessed January 23, 2003

21. UNICEF. *The State of the World's Children 2001.* Available at: http://www.unicef.org/sowc01/tables.pdf. Accessed February 1, 2003

22. Pan American Health Organization. World Health Organization. Jamaica Available at: http://www.paho.org/English/SHA/prfljam.htm. Accessed February 1, 2003

23. Joseph A. *Health-Caribbean: Cancer Deaths Rise as Lifestyle Changes.* Available at: http://www.oneworld.org/ips2/mar98/cancer.htm. Accessed February 1, 2003

24. Brathwaite C, Noble B. Are local foods too expensive for a healthy diet: urban obesity and rural poverty in Jamaica, two sides of the same coin? Presented at: Caribbean Health Research Council Annual Conference; April 2001; Kingston, Jamaica

25. Samuda P, Bushway A, Beecher G, et al. Nutrient content of commonly consumed Jamaican food and dishes. In: *TEKTRAN.* Beltsville, MD: United States Department of Agriculture, Agricultural Research Service; 1998

26. Relly J. *Caribbean AIDS Explosion Examined.* Available at: http://www.walterrodney.org/caribaids.htm. Accessed February 1, 2003

27. Ward M. *The Reproductive and Sexual Health of Jamaican Youth.* Washington, DC: Advocates for Youth; 2001

28. McCaw-Binns A, La Grenade J, Ashley D. Under-users of antenatal care: a comparison of non-attenders and late attenders for antenatal care, with early attenders. *Soc Sci Med.* 1995;40:1003–1012

29. Ragoobirsingh D, Lewis-Fuller E, Morrison E. The Jamaican diabetes survey: a protocol for the Caribbean. *Diabetes Care.* 1995;18:1277–1279

30. Himes J, Walker S, Williams S, Bennett F, Graham-McGregor S. A method to estimate prevalence of iron deficiency and iron deficiency anemia in adolescent Jamaican girls. *Am J Clin Nutr.* 1997;65:831–836

31. Hinman A, Hersh B, de Quadros C. Rational use of rubella vaccine for prevention of congenital rubella syndrome in the Americas [Spanish]. *Pan Am J Public Health.* 1998;4:156–160

32. Dreher M, Nugent K, Hudgins R. Prenatal marijuana exposure and neonatal outcomes in Jamaica: an ethnographic study. *Pediatrics.* 1994;93:254–260

33. Brady P. Ganja in Jamaica. *Cannabis Culture Magazine.* 1999;16:16–19

34. Huber A. Labor of love to improve birthing in the Caribbean. *Midwif Today.* 1999;51:45

35. Windsor-Richards K, Gillies P. Racial grouping and women's experience of giving birth in hospital. *Midwife.* 1988;4:171–176

36. Wilson L. Birth as a community experience: it can be achieved in a hospital! *Midwif Today.* 1997;41

37. Stern G, Kruckman L. Multi-disciplinary perspectives on postpartum depression: an anthropological critique. *Soc Sci Med.* 1983;17:1027–1041

38. Cunningham W, Segree W. Breast feeding promotion in an urban and a rural Jamaican hospital. *Soc Sci Med.* 1990;30:341–348

39. Potts M, Masho S. Sterilization, contraception and abortion: global issues for women. *Sex Marital Ther.* 1995;10:135–147

40. Sobo E. Abortion traditions in rural Jamaica. *Soc Sci Med.* 1996;42:495–508

41. Eggleston E, Jackson J, Hardee K. Sexual attitudes and behavior among young adolescents in Jamaica. *Int Fam Plann Perspect.* 1999;25:78–84, 91

42. Andrews A. *Bereavement Support Among Ethnic Minority Communities in Derby: A Report for Action for Bereavement Care.* Available at: http://www.multifaithnet.org/mfnopenaccess/research/online/drafts/aabereavement.htm. Accessed February 1, 2003

43. Barrett R. *Death and Dying in the Black Experience. Innovations in End-of-Life Care.* Available at: http://www.edc.org/lastacts. Accessed January 15, 2003

44. Modeste N, Caleb-Drayton V, Montgomery S. Barriers to early detection of breast cancer among women in a Caribbean population. *Pan Am J Public Health.* 1999;5:152–163

45. UniChef. *Caribbean Foods Glossary.* Available at: http://www.unichef.com/caribgloss.htm. Accessed January 15, 2003

46. Zarou G. Jamaican me hungry: Caribbean cuisine. *Digital Men.* Available at: http://www.digitalmen,com/09012000/debauchery/stories/deb090100mzjamaica.html. Accessed February 1, 2003

Further Reading

Barnes C. *Despite Legislation, Violence Against Women Continues.* Available at: http://www.hartford-hwp.com/archives/43/116.html)

Barnett B. *Case Study of the Women's Center of Jamaica Foundation Program for Adolescent Mothers.* Research Triangle Park, NC: Family Health International; 1996

Barrett L. *The Rastafarians.* Boston, MA: Beacon Press; 1997

Brunt M, Milbauer M. Health status and practices of urban Caribbean Latinos with diabetes mellitus. *Ethnicity Dis.* 1998;8:158–166

Campbell V, Caribbean Food and Nutrition Institute. *Caribbean foodways.* Kingston, Jamaica: Caribbean Food and Nutrition Institute and the Pan American Health Organization Pan American Sanitary Bureau Regional Office of the World health Organization; 1988

Cox C. Medical education, women's status, and medical issues' effect on women's health in the Caribbean. *Health Care Women Int.* 1997;18:383–393

DeSantis L, Thomas J, Sinnett K. Intergenerational concept of adolescent sexuality: implications for community-based reproductive health care with Haitian immigrants. *Public Health Nurs.* 1999;16:102–113

Eggleston E, Jackson J, Rountree W, Pan Z. Evaluation of a sexuality education program for young adolescents Jamaica. *Pan Am J Public Health.* 2000;7:102–112

Gaston M, Garry K. *African American and Caribbean Women.* Philadelphia, PA: Lippincott-Raven Publishing; 1997

Gerbase A, Toscano C, Titan S, Cuchi P, Gonzalez-Salvatierra R, Zacarias F. Sexually transmitted diseases in Latin America and the Caribbean. *Pan Am J Public Health.* 1999;6:362–370

Hardee K. *Reproductive Health Case Study: Jamaica.* Washington, DC: Futures Group International; 1998

Higginbottom G. Heart health-associated health beliefs and behaviours of adolescents of African and African Caribbean descent in two cities in the United Kingdom. *J Adv Nurs.* 2000;32:1234–1242

Higginbottom G. Black women and breast feeding: a UK investigation. *Health Visitor.* 1998;71:12–15

Keddie A. Psychological factors associated with teenage pregnancy in Jamaica. *Adolescence.* 1992;27:873–890

McFarlane C. *Reproductive Health Survey, Jamaica 1997, Final Report.* Atlanta, GA: Department of Health and Human Services, Centers for Disease Control and Prevention; 1998

Montgomery H. *Primitive Medicine in the Caribbean.* Available at: http://www.utdallas.edu/dept/sci_ed/montgomery/medicine.html

Morris L. *Contraceptive Prevalence Survey, Jamaica 1993.* Atlanta, GA: Department of Health and Human Services, Centers for Disease Control and Prevention; 1995

Rowe M. The women in Rastafari. *Caribbean Q.* 1980;26:13–21

Schwartz D. Caribbean folk beliefs and western psychiatry. *J Psychosoc Nurs Ment Health Serv.* 1985;23:26–30

Smith M. A midwife's journey to Jamaica. *Birth Issues.* 1997;6:17–20

Sobo E. Bodies, kin and flow: family planning in rural Jamaica. *Med Anthropol Q.* 1993;(1):50–73

Stone T. *Jamaican Women: Their Politics, Economics, Roles, and Religions.* Available at: http://debate.uvm.edu/dreadlibrary/stone.html

Taylor D. The meaning of dietary and occupational restrictions among the Island. *Carib Am Anthropol.* 1950;52:243–249

Torkington N. Black migrant women and health. *Womens Stud Int Forum.* 1995;18:153–158

Troy J. Nurse Turner, Jamaican midwife. *Midwif Today.* 2000;54:57

Internet Resources

http://www.eatethnic.com
>   Everything about ethnic foods and ingredients, international
>   holiday traditions, religious diets, regional customs, recipes,
>   fun food facts, and cultural nutrition resources.

http://www.nal.usda.gov/fnic/etext/000023.html
>   Ethnic food guide pyramids from the US Department of Agriculture.

http://www.paho.org/English/SHA/prfljam.htm
>   Pan American Health Organization summary of health in Jamaica.

http://www.agricola.umn.edu/foodways/african.pdf
>   African and Caribbean foodways.

http://www.kacike.org/cac-ike/Cultures.html
>   Caribbean Amerindian Centrelink (CAC) cultures and lifeways.

http://dmoz.org/Society/Ethnicity/Indigenous_People/Caribbean/
>   List of links to various topics related to the Caribbean population.

8
Perinatal Health Care Issues of Japanese Women

Sachiko Oshio and Shigeko Ito

According to the US Census Bureau, more than 1 million Japanese Americans and citizens of Japan were residing in the United States in 2000.[1] However, it must be underscored that Japanese Americans and Japanese citizens living in the United States are distinct groups with significantly different cultures and historic backgrounds. Most present-day Japanese Americans are the descendants of immigrants who came to the United States prior to the mid-1920s. Various federal and state laws and regulations were enacted from 1910 through 1924 prohibiting naturalization, land ownership, and immigration of Japanese nationals. The flow of immigrants from Japan was effectively cut off completely by 1924.[2] Consequently, most Japanese Americans of childbearing age are 2 to 4 generations removed from the original immigrants. While the *Issei* (the immigrant generation) and *Nisei* (the first American generation) historically experienced systematic discrimination that culminated in their internment experience during World War II, the current generation of Japanese Americans is quite assimilated into American culture. *Sansei* (the second American generation) or *Yonsei* (the third American generation) Japanese Americans typically do not speak Japanese, learn limited cultural customs of Japan from their parents, and hold their identity as Asian Americans rather than as Japanese.[2]

In 2002 312,936 Japanese citizens were estimated to be living in the United States and 113,233 were holding an immigrant visa to live in the United States permanently. Data provided by the Japanese

Ministry of Foreign Affairs indicated that while 3,493 of these people became US citizens that same year, most did not seek permanent residency status and would be returning to Japan within 2 to 5 years. More specifically, 199,703 Japanese citizens worked for Japanese companies and were accompanied by their families, and an estimated 87,157 were enrolled in American colleges and universities and/or English as a Second Language programs.[3,4] In contrast to culturally assimilated Japanese Americans, intercultural understanding by health care providers is necessary when caring for Japanese citizens who are in this country temporarily or who are newly arrived.

The Japanese tend to be more formal and reserved than Americans. Public touching or hugging is generally avoided, with bowing the most common form of greeting. However, touching between mothers and their young children is largely exempt from the general rule of public restraint. In the mother/child dyad, close physical proximity dominates the relationship, and physical contact is practiced freely and abundantly. In particular, Japanese mothers often use the term *skinship* to connote "close physical contact," a custom they value and perceive as a vital ingredient for nurturing relationships with their children.

Similar to their public restraint in touching, the Japanese also limit eye contact in social situations. Many may feel uncomfortable when being looked at and consider it rude to stare at someone in the face for a long time. In social conversations, they may glance at the other person but generally avoid prolonged direct eye contact, particularly with an authority figure. However, it is considered appropriate for health care providers to directly look at their patients while tending to them.

Gender of the health care provider is not a major issue. Although the presence of a female nurse is reassuring for Japanese women, it is not culturally specified. While either gender for physician is likely to be accepted, they are not familiar with male midwives. To many Japanese, "yes" and "no" can be confusing. In their native language, "yes" *(hai)* simply means "I hear you" or "I understand what you are saying." If a negative question is asked, they might very well answer "Yes," meaning, for instance, "That's right, I don't," which to them is the same as saying "No, I don't." Such miscommunication can be avoided by carefully rephrasing the question when in doubt. Japanese also value social harmony and favor agreement. Even when they know that their answer is clearly no, they have difficulty directly answering "No," and may display hesitation and discomfort in communicating a negative response.

The following discussion attempts to capture the cultural characteristics of contemporary Japanese in America. As with any cultural group, there are individual, regional, and generational variations that affect acculturation into the United States. Addressing these differences is beyond the scope of this chapter, and generalizations drawn here should be taken with such a perspective in mind.

Health and Illness

Japan has the longest life expectancy at birth among all of the industrialized nations[5] and its perinatal mortality rate of 2 deaths per 1,000 births in 2000[6] was less than one third of that reported for the United States (6.9 deaths per 1,000 births).[7] Given the more favorable health indices of Japan, unfamiliar American technologies tend to be regarded as inferior by some Japanese, despite the fact that high-tech medical equipment and interventions as well as pharmacologic regimens have been very well accepted in Japan. Complementary health care practices such as Chinese herbal medicine, acupuncture, and acupressure have long coexisted with Western medicine in Japan; together both modalities have become well integrated into the Japanese mainstream.

Pregnancy/Prenatal Care

Pregnancy and childbearing are taken very seriously in Japan. There are many statutes that protect pregnant women and provide for maternity leave before and after birth. For example, an additional law was recently enacted that allows either parent to take an unpaid parental leave for up to 1 year. It is also illegal for a company to fire a woman because of pregnancy. In addition to regular prenatal care and extended postpartum hospital stays (5–10 days), first-time mothers also receive home visits from public health nurses.

Cut off from their accustomed support systems, pregnant Japanese women may feel isolated and somewhat helpless in the United States. Language barriers as well as unfamiliarity with American customs, the health care system, and the availability of community resources are all likely to contribute to their anxiety. Because Japanese women come from a culture where passivity is favored,[8] many Japanese women may not seek help actively; rather, they might expect others to initiate help without making any request on their own behalf.

A *Maternal Health Handbook* is issued to every pregnant woman by the local government in Japan. The pregnant woman brings her handbook *(Boshi Kenkou Techo)* to every prenatal visit, and all of the pertinent clinical information is recorded there. This handbook belongs to the baby, and a cumulative summary of all of the essential health information from conception through school age becomes the child's health record. Some Japanese women may have a handbook already started by the time they begin prenatal care in the United States and may even obtain an English version so that American health care providers can make entries in their books. They will appreciate the cooperation of American health care providers in maintaining these records.

Ultrasound is used frequently in Japan. Some pregnant women may express dissatisfaction about not having sonograms done at every prenatal visit[9] and may be surprised to learn that their American insurance companies pay only for medically necessary sonograms. However, prenatal screening by serum markers is not as commonly used in Japan as in the United States. Consequently, many would decline maternal serum alphafetoprotein (MSAFP) testing and associated tests.

It is estimated that 342,000 pregnancies were terminated in 2001, which amounts to one third of the number of births in Japan that year (1.2 million).[10] Abortion may be included in the discussion of options if prenatal testing reveals anomalies.

Many Japanese in the United States incorporate traditional Japanese foods into their daily diet along with regular American foods. The typical Japanese meal consists of a bowl of white rice, a bowl of miso (salted and fermented soybean paste) soup, some kind of meat or fish dish, pickled vegetables, and warm or cold vegetable dishes on the side. Some of the traditional foods that are recommended during pregnancy are presented in Table 8-1.

Salt restriction is commonly recommended in Japan for the purpose of preventing excessive edema and high blood pressure during pregnancy, particularly because traditional Japanese foods tend to be high in salt. Pregnant Japanese women living in the United States may carry over the practice of reducing their salt intake. This is usually accomplished by using low sodium soy sauce, limiting the amount of miso soup (and by eating the cooked vegetables in the soup and leaving the salty liquid), and avoiding highly salted pickles, fish, and

Table 8-1
Food Preferences of Pregnant Japanese Women

For Increased Intake Of	Recommended Food
Calcium	*Tofu,* shiba-ebi (dried small shrimp), *chirimen-jako* (steamed and dried small fish), *hijiki* (dried seaweed)
Iron	Clams, various greens *(daikon green, komatsuna, shungiku,* etc), seaweed
Vitamins	Cooked spinach, broccoli, seaweed, fruits, sesame seeds
Protein	*Tofu* (raw, cooked, dried, fried, mixed with fish, etc), cooked soybeans, fish (dried, cooked, broiled), bean sprouts, shellfish

fish roe. The use of citrus vinegar *(ponzu, yuzu)* in place of soy sauce is often effective in reducing salt intake.

Many Japanese pregnant women are concerned and confused about higher weight gain recommendations in the United States (25–35 lbs),[11] compared with those made in Japan (8–10 kg, or 17.5–22 lbs).[12] To make matters worse, many Japanese women have low body mass index (BMI) compared with American women, and American health care providers may recommend the higher end of pregnancy weight gain scale for them based on the recommendation by the Institute of Medicine for underweight pregnant women. Thus while their weight gain is considered to be insufficient by American medical practitioners, they themselves may be concerned that they have far exceeded the safe weight gain recommendations.

Counter to popular beliefs about Japanese food being low in calories, many dishes are deep fried and high in calories. For example, tempura (deep fried fish and vegetables), *Katsu* (deep-fried pork), and *Korokke* (croquettes) are very common daily dishes for Japanese. Advice on cutting down fat intake would be welcomed by those women struggling to stay within the ideal weight gain recommendations while maintaining good nutrition.

Pregnant women are often reminded about the harm of "being chilled" *(hieru)*. "Chilling" is believed to cause the common cold, diarrhea, and other ailments that may harm the pregnancy or fetus. Women are cautioned against eating large quantities of raw vegetables and fruits, such as watermelon, because they may cause abdominal chilling. Warm socks are worn even during the hot season because cold feet are supposed to be bad for the uterus and fetus. Many pregnant women become very cautious about the use of air conditioners for fear of causing harm to the fetus.

Tai-kyou (teaching while in the womb) is an important concept in Asian countries. It is roughly interpreted in Japan as "taking care of the fetus through the attention of pregnant women to their own mental and physical health." Anything that would disturb a pregnant woman's mental or physical status is not good for *Tai-kyou*. It is feared that there might be some unexpected effect on the fetus if the pregnant woman is exposed to unpleasant feelings or if her attitude toward life is negative. Some take it further and listen to classical music, meditate, eat special foods, and avoid stressful events, hoping for positive effects on the fetus.

Fukutai, or *Haraobi,* is a special maternity sash worn by pregnant women. Different regional traditions dictate slightly different methods, but the most common custom is to apply a plain white cotton sash on the Day of the Dog, according to the Chinese calendar around the fifth month of pregnancy. The Chinese calendar assigns 1 of the 12 animals and 4 earthly elements to each day, and the Day of the Dog appears every 12 days. Dogs are believed to be very fertile and have easy births; thus applying the sash on the Day of the Dog is supposed to ensure the woman a safe birth. Maternity sashes also serve as protective garments for pregnant women by preventing the pregnant abdomen from getting chilled and by giving support to abdominal muscles.

Some women obtain an amulet *(Omamori)* for an easy and safe birth *(An-Zan)* from a *Shinto* shrine. It is typically placed in a red pouch, and often worn like a necklace under clothing throughout the pregnancy. Family members or friends may make a special trip to the shrine and obtain this amulet with *Shinto* blessings for the pregnant woman living abroad. Health care providers in the United States may see it worn by women during labor. Some amulets contain a few grains of rice and a small piece of paper with a special prayer written on it. Women in labor are supposed to swallow those items to make the amulet effective.

Japanese fathers are beginning to get involved in pregnancy and birth. Although gender role differentiation has started to weaken in recent years, the pattern of involvement in pregnancy, birth, and child care is somewhat different from that of American men. A survey published in 2001 revealed that activities such as bathing a baby and changing diapers are becoming more common among younger Japanese men.[13] However, direct participation by fathers in childbirth preparation classes and their presence at birth is still estimated to be only about 30% in Japan.[14]

Prenatal breast and nipple massages are often recommended in Japan. Women are taught to lift up and move the bases of both breasts in different directions several times a day starting in midpregnancy to enhance circulation, and to roll the nipples between the fingers for better nipple protrusion, cleaning the clogged ducts, and "toughening" the nipple skin.[15] Japanese women may ask about the specifics of preparing their breasts during prenatal care in the United States and may feel discouraged by the inadequate guidance they receive. American health care providers might invoke the help of female family members in securing Japanese instructional books or videos for the woman's use.

Sexual intercourse is usually recommended to be limited during the last trimester, and in some cases, until after 7 weeks' gestation. Many pregnancy guidebooks recommend shallow penetration, slow easy movements, and the use of a condom so that the pregnancy is not disturbed.

Labor and Delivery

Japanese hospitals do no commonly allow or encourage the attendance of the husband at the birth. Many men also regard labor and birth as the women's domain and feel out of place. When a Japanese wife is having a baby in the United States, the husband may feel obligated to attend the birth due to American cultural expectations and for the practicality of being an interpreter for his wife. These husbands typically do not see themselves as major supporters in labor and, consequently, do not prepare themselves for coaching roles. Many Japanese women who give birth in the United States invite their own mothers from Japan to be with them.

Japanese women tend to be less expressive of their pain or their need for support compared with American women. Coming from a culture where others are supposed to be empathetic and able to anticipate their needs, Japanese women are not used to being asked what they want. They are accustomed to having other people anticipate their needs and make decisions for them.

Food intake during labor is not restricted in Japan; it is encouraged to keep up the woman's energy. Ambulation is not commonly encouraged, and traditional delivery tables with lithotomy stirrups are often used. Most Japanese women go through labor naturally, without medication. However, some Japanese women in the United States may expect to have epidural anesthesia because they believe that is how childbirth is conducted in this country.

Midwives were the main care providers for pregnant women in Japan until the American occupation, when the US army discouraged the traditional practices of midwifery and out-of-hospital births. Currently, 99.9% of births occur in institutions and are attended by obstetricians with midwives assuming auxiliary roles. Midwives in Japanese hospitals function just like obstetric nurses in the United States. Thus Japanese women may be surprised to learn that nurses on American labor units are not midwives. They may also have difficulty understanding the independent practice of nurse-midwives in the United States because there is no such comparable midwifery role in Japan. Although the presence of a female nurse is reassuring for Japanese women, it is not culturally specified. While either gender for physician is likely to be accepted, they are not familiar with male midwives.

Postpartum and Newborn Care

Japanese mothers tend to look to midwives and nurses for expert advice in every aspect of self-care and baby care. In Japan, most mothers stay in the hospital for 5 to 10 days. Extensive teaching and careful monitoring of maternal recovery and the infant's condition are provided and activities are highly proscribed. For example, taking a shower is not usually allowed until the second or third day, and shampooing the hair is further delayed. The traditional custom of avoiding water is probably based on the fear of being "chilled" and also because of concerns about fainting. Doctors routinely perform an examination on the fifth day postpartum, and episiotomy stitches are removed at that time if nonabsorbable sutures are used. A Japanese woman who gives birth in the United States may be unsure of what to expect when no one tells her when the stitches will be removed or when she can shampoo her hair.

Breastfeeding is highly controlled in Japanese hospitals. The value of colostrum is not widely appreciated, and breastfeeding is often not initiated until the second day postpartum. Many Japanese hospitals use communal breastfeeding rooms, where mothers are summoned every 4 hours to nurse their babies. Babies are weighed before and after nursing, and supplemental formula or expressed milk is provided if the intake is not sufficient. Japanese women who breastfeed in the United States may express anxiety over not knowing the exact intake of the infant and may request supplementation. The value of colostrum and the relationship between demand feeding and breast milk supply should be explained to them.

Postpartum breast massage by professionals is a thriving business in Japan. Some midwives are certified in the *Oketani* method (named after a renowned midwife who started this therapy) and provide massage services for women with breastfeeding problems. The technique is carefully guarded, and only a limited number of people are certified. The purpose of the massage is to improve circulation, increase milk production, improve the quality of the milk, prevent clogged ducts, and remove any existing blockage.[16] Lactation consultants may be able to suggest alternative ways of attaining these same goals. According to 1997 data,[17] the rate of breastfeeding (including mixed feeding) at 1 month postpartum in Japan was 90.9%. This compares favorably with the 1998 rate for the United States, which was 64% at the time of hospital discharge.[18]

Sticky rice and white fish are recommended for nursing mothers in Japan. Miso soup with shellfish is also believed to increase milk production. Ceremonial feeding (*Okuizome* [pretending only]) of rice and fish by an elder relative is observed when the baby is about 100 days old and represents a wish for a plentiful food supply for the baby's lifetime. This is just a ceremony, and the real introduction of solids will not happen until the fifth month.

Some Japanese parents may feel the American custom of selecting a baby's name before the birth to be too hasty. Traditionally, babies are named on the seventh day with ceremonial writing of the name with *sumi* ink on white paper. The name is displayed in a prominent place in the house and is taken down when the birth certificate is officially submitted to the municipal office 2 weeks after birth. Although middle names are not recognized in Japan, some Japanese choose to give their babies a Western middle name solely for the American birth certificate.

Bathing the baby in a tub is accepted and encouraged in Japan, even while the umbilical cord is attached. The umbilical cord, believed to have a special connection to a higher power or the world beyond this life, was preserved in a special wooden box in the past. This custom has declined and is not commonly practiced anymore. Circumcisions, either male or female, are not practiced in Japan. Parents present their baby in ceremonial garb to a *Shinto* shrine at 1 month of age. Parents and both sets of grandparents express thanks to the *Shinto* god for the baby's safe passage into this world and wish for health and safety throughout the baby's life.

Cosleeping remains a widely accepted norm in Japan, and it is not uncommon to find the mother (or both parents) sharing the bed with a child beyond the age of 3 years. Matsuda,[19] a Japanese child care expert who is often referred to as the Japanese version of Dr Spock, contends that cosleeping is natural and has no long-term harmful effects. Japanese women may feel surprised about the strong opposition to this practice by some Americans.

Family Planning

Sexual activity is usually resumed after the postpartum examination at 4 to 6 weeks. The most common contraceptive used in Japan is the condom. Oral contraceptive pills became legal in Japan for the first time in late 1999. However, many Japanese women consider oral contraceptives to be dangerous if continued more than 1 or 2 years. Intrauterine devices (IUDs) and diaphragms are acceptable family planning methods, although used much less frequently than condoms.

Safe and legal abortion services are easily obtained in Japan at obstetricians' offices. Most of the abortions are performed for married couples because of contraceptive failures.

Bioethical Dilemmas

Paternalistic attitudes of medical professionals toward their patients are very common in Japan, and many Japanese parents expect the same from the American health care providers. Some patients find making choices burdensome, and they rely on their health care providers to make the best decisions for them. In addition, when language barriers exist, Japanese women may hesitate to ask for clarifications and/or to discuss matters thoroughly. For example, a study conducted in Pennsylvania quoted one Japanese woman as stating, "I did not fully understand the physician's explanation. Therefore, I usually followed his suggestions without deciding by myself even though he showed me several alternatives."[9]

This lack of full involvement in decision making may occasionally result in outcomes for which they did not consent with full understanding. A few mothers stated that they did not understand what was to be done to their sons when they went along with their American husband's wish to have their sons circumcised. Because circumcisions

are not done in Japan, they did not have an accurate understanding
of the procedure or the consequences from it, and were later very
surprised and saddened by the extent of the injury sustained by
their sons.

There are several additional contributing factors that encourage
the passivity of Japanese patients. One is the cultural pattern of relating to each other. It is very common for Japanese to rely on others
to look after them when they are in stressful situations. This type of
mutual dependency is called *amae*[20]; it discourages a person from
actively asserting their own preferences or opinion. One may also
have to consider that their sense of self-efficacy as an autonomous
adult is usually eroded to a certain degree, and that may prevent them
from fully participating in medical decision making. Living in a foreign country, they find that their highly developed sense of social
appropriateness, age-old common sense, and sophisticated usage
of native language are all quite useless.

Death/Burial Rites

In Japan, most death and funeral rites follow the Buddhist tradition,
with regional and local variations in specific practices. Typically, the
day after someone dies, the family and relatives hold a wakelike ritual
called tsuya (literally translated as "throughout the night") during the
night before the funeral. The funeral, which is more public, is usually
held the day after the death. Afterward, the family and close friends
accompany the deceased to a crematorium and stay while the body is
being cremated. Once the cremation is completed, the bones and ashes
are brought out, and the family and friends line up in pairs to pick up
the bones; by using 2 pair of long chopsticks, they place one piece at
a time into an urn. Some families bring the urn home and keep it on
an altar for 49 days, while other families place it in the cemetery right
after the cremation. In Buddhism, it is believed that the spirit remains
with the family for 49 days, after which each spirit transcends into a
Buddha. The spirits of the departed as well as ancestors are believed

to return to visit their descendants for 1 week each summer (O-Bon), during which time additional memorial services are held. Not having family and traditional Japanese undertakers to guide them through the complicated ritual, some families defer the ritual until they get back to Japan to turn the ashes into their ancestral grave.

There are special Buddhas called *mizuko,* which represent any fetus that never became a baby, including one that was aborted, miscarried, or stillborn. *Mizuko* literally means "water child," and no funeral services are held for them. However, women may pay a neighborhood temple to make a memorial statue *(mizuko jizo)* to commemorate the lost child.[21] Often a number of these statues in the image of serene-faced small Buddhas are grouped together in a temple garden; generally, they do not bear names of either the child or the mother. Monks of the temple will pray for those unborn children, and people will show respect by pouring water on the statues as they pass by them. Today, one can purchase a *mizuko jizo* and related services over the Internet.

Every Japanese Woman Is Unique

Given the existence of different cultural assumptions, customs, and expectations regarding health and illness among Japanese people, it is reasonable to anticipate some degree of misunderstanding, confusion, or conflict between US health care professionals and their Japanese clients. American health care providers need to keep in mind that such disparities are not merely caused by the language barrier, but may also arise from different cultural factors.[9]

Some Japanese women assimilate into American culture easily, while others limit their association to close-knit Japanese expatriates only. Some maintain the traditional role of stoic, dedicated wives, yet others choose to come to the United States for the freedom accorded to the women in this country. Their comfort level in the American health care system varies accordingly. Assessing each woman's needs individually is always a sensible approach.

Perinatal Health Care Issues of Japanese Women: Key Highlights

Demographic/Psychosocial/Spiritual Characteristics

- Japan has the longest life expectancy at birth among all of the industrialized nations and had a perinatal mortality rate of 2 deaths per 1,000 births in 2000.
- 1 million Japanese Americans and citizens of Japan were residing in the United States in 2000.
- Japanese Americans and Japanese citizens living in the United States are distinct groups with significantly different cultures and historic backgrounds.
- Japanese Americans typically do not speak Japanese, learn limited cultural customs of Japan from their parents, and hold their identity as Asian Americans rather than as Japanese.
- In the Japanese language, "yes" *(hai)* simply means "I hear you" or "I understand what you are saying" and does not necessarily mean "Yes, I do," "Yes, I am," or "Yes, it is."
- Touching or hugging is minimal; bowing, the most common form of greeting, does not involve touching.
- Japanese women are typically reserved and speak softly.
- Although eye contact is usually avoided, it is culturally acceptable for health care providers to look directly at Japanese patients while tending to them.
- Although the presence of a female nurse is reassuring for Japanese women, it is not culturally specified. Either gender for physician is likely to be accepted.

Prenatal Care

- The *Maternal Health Handbook* is maintained from conception to school age, summarizing all of the essential health information for the child. Every prenatal visit is entered into this record.

- A weight gain recommendation in the United States (25–35 lbs) is higher compared with that of Japanese recommendations (17.5–22 lbs).
- Prenatal breast and nipple massages are often recommended in Japan.
- *Tai-kyou* is the practice of "taking care of the fetus through the attention of a pregnant woman to her own mental and physical health." Anything that would disturb a pregnant woman's mental or physical status is not good for *Tai-kyou.*
- *Fukutai,* or *Haraobi,* a special maternity sash, is worn by pregnant women to provide abdominal support and protection from "chilling."

Prenatal Testing
- Pregnant women may expect to have many ultrasounds, but may not be familiar with MSAFP and related testings.

Pregnancy Diet
- Some women may avoid raw vegetables and fruits that may cause abdominal chilling.
- Tofu, fish, dried seafoods, various Asian green vegetables, and sesame seeds are among the main sources of protein, vitamins, and minerals.

Pregnancy-Related Beliefs/Taboos
- Wearing the *Fukutai,* or *Haraobi,* on the Day of the Dog is supposed to ensure a safe birth.
- It is feared that there might be some unexpected effect on the fetus if the pregnant woman is exposed to unpleasant feelings or if her attitude toward life is negative.
- "Chilling" is believed to cause the common cold, diarrhea, and other ailments that may harm the pregnancy or fetus.
- Some women place an amulet *(Omamori)* in a red pouch and wear it like a necklace under clothing throughout the pregnancy for an easy and safe birth *(An-Zan).*

Labor and Delivery

- Analgesia and anesthesia are usually not administered during labor or birth in Japan. Many desire an epidural in the United States because it is perceived as the American way.
- Postpartum analgesia is not commonly administered.
- Many are not familiar with options other than the lithotomy position for birth.
- The hospital is the most common place for birth.
- Ambulation during labor is not routinely allowed in Japan.
- Eating unrestricted during labor is encouraged in Japan.
- Fathers may not be comfortable in the support role. The mother of the laboring woman sometimes assumes the support role.

Postpartum Care

- Shampooing hair and bathing are sometimes avoided for several days postpartum due to the traditional custom of avoiding the chilling effects of water.

Postpartum Diet

- Miso soup with shellfish is believed to increase milk production.
- See Pregnancy Diet

Neonatal Care

- Circumcision is not practiced in Japan.
- Babies are named on the seventh day in Japan. Ceremonial writing of the name with *sumi* ink on a white paper is performed.
- Parents present their baby in ceremonial garb to a *Shinto* shrine at 1 month of age.
- A ceremonial feeding of fish by an elder relative is observed when the baby is about 100 days old.
- Many practice breastfeeding and bottle-feeding soon after the birth.
- Cosleeping with mother and family is common up to toddler age.

Breastfeeding/Breast Care

- Breast massage to increase the quantity and improve the quality of milk by a specialist is commonly practiced in Japan.

Family Involvement

- Major decisions are often made by Japanese husbands.
- About 30% of husbands are present at birth in Japan; they participate more in the United States, partly functioning as interpreters for their wives.
- Other children are not usually present at the birth in Japan. However, the family may bring older siblings to the birth if the family does not have child care arrangements in the United States.

Pregnancy Termination/Miscarriage

- Pregnancy termination is usually an acceptable option for an undesirable pregnancy.

Family Planning

- The most common contraceptive method used in Japan is the condom.
- Oral contraceptive pills, IUDs, and the diaphragm are also acceptable for family planning.

Bioethical Dilemmas

- Medical professionals are expected to know what is best for the woman, and some families may find decision making to be too burdensome.

Death/Burial Rites

- Most death/funeral rites follow the Buddhist tradition. Some families defer rituals until after they return to Japan due to the lack of proper support in the United States.
- The spirit is believed to remain with the family for 49 days, after which it transcends into a Buddha. The spirits of the departed are believed to return to visit their descendants for 1 week each summer (O-Bon), during which time additional memorial services are held.

- Special Buddhas, called *Mizuko,* represent any fetus that never became a baby, including one that was aborted, miscarried, or stillborn. There are no funeral services for such "water children," but statues honoring them are often found in Buddhist temples.

References

1. US Census Bureau. *2000 Census of Population and Housing, Asian Population Detailed Group Table.* Available at: http://www.census.gov/ prod/2002pubs/c2kbr01-16.pdf. Accessed February 1, 2003
2. Takezawa Y. Breaking the silence: redress and Japanese American ethnicity. In: Sanjek R, ed. *Anthropology of Contemporary Issues.* Ithaca, NY: Cornell University Press; 1995
3. Ministry of Foreign Affairs of Japan. *Number of Japanese Living Abroad by Country (As of 10/01/2002).* Available at: http://www.mofa.go.jp/mofaj/ toko/tokei/hojin/02/2.html#3. Accessed February 1, 2003
4. Ministry of Foreign Affairs of Japan. *Japanese Students Overseas (1983– 2000).* Available at: http://jin.jcic.or.jp/stat/stats/16EDU62.html. Accessed February 1, 2003
5. Ministry of Health, Labour and Welfare of Japan. *Abridged Life Table (July 31, 2001).* Available at: http://www.jinjapan.org/stat/stats/ 02VIT25.html. Accessed February 1, 2003
6. Ministry of Health, Labour and Welfare of Japan. *Infant, Newborn, and Perinatal Mortality Table (1947–2000).* Available at: http://www.gender.go.jp/ sabetsu/5th_report/toukei/1213.pdf. Accessed February 1, 2003
7. Centers for Disease Control and Prevention. Infant mortality. *Natl Vital Stat Rep.* 2002;50
8. Ito M, Sharts-Hopko N. Japanese women's experience of childbirth in the United States. *Health Care Women Int.* 2002;23:666–667
9. Yeo S, Fetters M, Maeda Y. Japanese couples' childbirth experiences in Michigan: implications for care. *Birth.* 2000;27:191–198
10. Ministry of Health, Labour and Welfare of Japan. *Vital Statistics: Births.* Available at: http://www.jinjapan.org/stat/stats/02VIT11.html. Accessed February 1, 2003
11. Institute of Medicine. *Nutrition During Pregnancy: Part I Weight Gain, Part II Nutritional Supplement.* Washington, DC: National Academy Press; 1990
12. Shufu no Tomo. *Shussan Hyakka [Encyclopedia of Birth].* Tokyo, Japan: Shufu no Tomo Co. Ltd; 1993

13. Igarashi H, Iijima S. Fathers' modes of thinking and behavior in childcare. *Yamanashi Idai Kiyou.* 2001;18:89–93

14. Kawai R. *Osan Erabi Manual [How to Choose Your Birth Experiences].* Tokyo, Japan: Nobunkyo; 2000

15. Fujimori K. *Nyubo Jiko Kanri [Practice of Self-Management of Breast Care].* Tokyo, Japan: Medica Publishing; 1996

16. Pearse J. Breast-feeding practices in Japan. *Midwives Chronicle.* 1990:310–314

17. Ministry of Health, Labour and Welfare of Japan. *Heisei 7 nen nyuuyouji eiyou cyousa kekka [Infant Dietary Intake Survey of 1997].* Available at: http://www1.mhlw.go.jp/houdou/0902/h0214-1.html. Accessed February 1, 2003

18. US Department of Health and Human Services. *Healthy People 2010: Understanding and Improving Health.* 2nd ed. Washington, DC: US Government Printing Office; 2000. Available at: http://www.healthypeople.gov/document/html/tracking/od16.htm#breastfeeding. Accessed February 1, 2003

19. Matsuda M. *Nihonshiki Ikujihou.* Tokyo, Japan: Kodansha; 1973

20. Doi T. Some thoughts on helplessness and the desire to be loved. *Psychiatry.* 1963;26:266–272

21. La Fleur WR. *Liquid Life: Abortion and Buddhism in Japan.* Princeton, NJ: Princeton University Press; 1944

Further Reading/Viewing

Wynd, O. *The Ginger Tree.* New York, NY: Harper Perennial; 1990

O-soshiki (The Funeral). A film directed by Itami Juzo, 1985 Wellspring

9
Perinatal Health Care Issues of Jewish Women

Ellen Shuzman

Judaism is both a religion and an ethnic identity. It celebrates life and procreation. While the Jewish male is commanded to "be fruitful and multiply," the Jewish female is taught that her life is centered around marriage and raising a family. Even the Jewish clergy (rabbis) are expected to marry and procreate. Jews believe that there is one almighty God and that God is spiritual and moral and demands moral and ethical behavior. Central to the Jewish belief is that God communicated how one should live through the 10 commandments.

The term *Jew* historically has been synonymous with Hebrew and/or Israelite.[1] Jews believe that they are descendants of the Bible's Abraham, also called Hebrew. Israel, a grandson of Abraham, and his descendants became known as the Children of Israel, or the Israelite People. The term *Jew* comes from Judah, the son of Israel, and also the name of the tribe of his descendants. Today the people are called *Jewish,* their language *Hebrew,* and their faith *Judaism.*[1]

In biblical times Jews lived in the land of Canaan, which was later called Israel. By 515 BC, however, many Jews left that land and settled in a variety of countries to escape the dangers of constant war and the presence of foreign rulers. Thus contemporary Israel is considered the homeland of all Jews, even though the Jewish people, as an ethnic group, have immigrated there from many countries. Jews of eastern European descent are called *Ashkenazim,* while those from the Mediterranean and other regions are called *Sephardim.* Many customs and practices surrounding daily Jewish life are observed differently by the descendants of each group.[2,3] American Jews are predominantly of Ashkenazic descent.

Although Hebrew is the official language of Judaism, Jews live in all parts of the world and speak a variety of languages. Yiddish, a dialect based on German, is spoken by Jews from Eastern Europe; when written, it uses Hebrew characters. In the early 1900s European Jews brought Yiddish to the United States. Today it is less widely spoken, but many words, such as *yenta* and *chutzpah,* have become part of the English vernacular.

Regardless of where they exist, all synagogues (Jewish houses of worship) have prayers written in Hebrew, and many use the same melodies for many of the prayers, so that any Jew from any part of the world can join in prayer. Because the history of the Jewish people is so tied in with religious persecution and exile from their homelands, affiliation and kinship with other Jews is important. The feeling of kinship felt by Jewish people of varying nationalities is partly perpetuated through their common language as well as religious and cultural practices.

The Jewish bible is composed of 3 parts: the *Torah* (the 5 books of Moses), the *Nevi'im,* and the *Ketuvim* (the Psalms, Proverbs, and other books). The *Torah* contains all of the Jewish beliefs, practices, and writing that give guidance and instruction on how to live and behave.[1] The *Nevi'im* and *Ketuvim* are what non-Jews refer to as the Old Testament. The *Talmud* is a collection of laws and commentary on the *Torah.*[4,5]

To further clarify Jewish law, the *Halachah* has evolved.[1,4–6] This collection of rabbinical decisions applies Jewish law to specific day-to-day situations and deals with ethical obligations, religious duties, and a commitment to the commandments.[1,5] As medical technology advances, the rabbis are challenged with making decisions as to whether new technology and procedures are permissible or if they violate Jewish law. Rabbinical decisions are communicated in the *Halachah.*[1,5]

Today Judaism has 3 levels of practice: Orthodox, Conservative, and Reform. The Orthodox Jew adheres most strictly to the *Torah* and the *Halachah;* the Conservative Jew is less strict in interpreting the *Torah* and following the *Halachah;* the Reform Jew is liberal in practice. In addition to these 3 levels of practicing Judaism, there are numerous individual variations. For example, it is not unusual for a Jewish home to be kosher (in accord with Jewish dietary laws); yet the family may eat in non-kosher restaurants. Because Orthodox Jews are the most strict in their adherence to the *Torah* and *Halachah,* much of the discussion in this chapter will focus on their particular level of practice.

Prayers are an essential component of daily life for the observant Jew. The Orthodox Jew will recite daily prayers 3 times a day. Although men are obligated to arrange their daily schedules so that prayers may be said within specific time frames and to attend prayer services, the rules for women are flexible. Women are required to pray, but they can do so at any time and not within a formal service. Women are expected to focus first on their roles of wife and mother. However, whenever prayers are said they are not to be interrupted or said in haste or without meaning.

The Jewish Sabbath is extremely important to observant Jews. Many of the customs, laws, and obligations associated with the Sabbath are also observed during the major Jewish holy days. The Sabbath begins on Friday evening at sundown and continues through until sunset on Saturday evening. It is a day in which the Jews rest and participate in spiritual activities that include attending synagogue services, spending time with family, studying the *Torah,* and eating traditional foods. On Friday evenings at sundown, married women and single adults light special candles, after which the customs of the Sabbath begin. Prior to eating any meals on the Sabbath, a blessing known as *Kiddush* is recited over the wine or juice. The Sabbath ends with a service called the *Havdala* ceremony, in which blessings are said over wine, spices, and candle lighting.

Many of the Sabbath customs have evolved from the fact that the main purpose of the Sabbath is to replenish or refresh the body and soul of the Jew. Accordingly, on the Sabbath, it is customary for the Orthodox Jew, and for many Conservative Jews, to refrain from work-related activities including, but not limited to, operating electrically run appliances, lights, or equipment; riding in elevators or cars; turning on a flame or striking a match; and writing, tearing, cutting, or sewing. These customs are also observed on the major holy days.

Many Jewish holy days require adults to refrain from eating or drinking for a specified period of time. Fasting on 2 major holy days, Yom Kippur (the Day of Atonement) and Tisha B'Av, begins at sunset of the holy day and continues for 25 hours. Some minor holy days require that fasting begin at dawn and end at sundown. Adults of all levels of Judaism are most likely to fast on Yom Kippur; Orthodox and other Jews, to a lesser extent, will fast on the other holy days.

Judaism places a strong value on family purity. Marriage bonds between a man and a woman are viewed as an opportunity to bring holiness to one's life.[7] Intimacy and love are intricately woven into family purity. Intimate, sexual relations between a man and a woman are considered a blessing and a reflection of God's presence.[7] Celibacy in marriage is a sign of disrespect for God's plans.[5] Intercourse is not just for procreation but for the sexual pleasure of the woman and the man[4]; however, the *Torah* stresses that it must be an act of intimacy and reflect love and respect. To this end, the *Torah* and the *Halachah* provide the laws of *niddah* to maintain family purity.

The laws of *niddah* are a set of rules that primarily focus on restrictions in the wife's sexual availability.[4,5,7,8] A woman is considered to be impure, or *niddah,* whenever she menstruates or experiences uterine bleeding. During the state of *niddah,* the husband and wife are not permitted to have any physical contact.

Indirect contact, such as the husband picking up a belonging of his wife's or the wife handing an object to her husband, is prohibited. The *niddah* state exists for at least 12 days when a woman has menstruated, including the actual days for the menstrual period followed by 7 days of no sign of bleeding. If bleeding occurs following a gynecologic examination and the health care practitioner cannot say with 100% certainty that the blood is not uterine, the woman is considered *niddah.* To restore a state of purity, the woman takes a ritual bath called a *mikvah.*[1,9] Sexual intercourse is prohibited until after this cleansing. The *mikvah* cannot be any body of water; the tub must be at least 24 cubic feet[8] and contain at least 191 gallons of natural water.[9] It may be located in a synagogue or in a freestanding building.

The *Halachah* stresses that there should be modesty in every aspect of one's life and in relationships with others. Unduly exposing a part of the body that is usually covered is improper. Orthodox men and women often wear long-sleeved clothing and head coverings throughout the day. When in the synagogue, the Conservative male, and to a lesser extent the Reform male, will wear a skullcap, also called a *yarmulke* in Yiddish and a *kipa* in Hebrew. The *Hasidim,* a group of Orthodox Jews, dress and groom in a manner that more overtly sets them apart from mainstream America. Specifically, *Hasidic* married women wear wigs or other head coverings for modesty and to communicate their marital status.[9] *Hasidic* men have beards and long sideburns, cover their heads with a skullcap or hat, and typically wear dark clothing.

The laws of *kashrut,* the Hebrew word for the kosher, are the dietary rules governing what the observant Jew can eat and what utensils may be used. All vegetables and fish that have fins and scales are considered kosher. Meat from an animal that has fully split hooves, chews cud, and has been ritually slaughtered by an authorized kosher butcher is also considered kosher but needs to be further soaked for 30 minutes and then salted for 1 hour.

In accordance with the laws of *kashrut,* a Jew will not eat meat and dairy products at the same time. After a meat meal, it is mandated to wait as long as 6 hours before ingesting dairy products. The waiting period for eating meat after dairy is at least 30 minutes, but can be longer depending on the dairy product. Furthermore, porous dishes and utensils may not be used for meat and dairy products. Most kosher homes will have 2 sets of dishes, pots, pans, and utensils, one set for meat and one for dairy. Many authorities support the use of one set of glass dishes for either meat or dairy claiming that glass is nonporous. Most kosher homes will also have another set of pots, pans, utensils, and some neutral dishes, labeled *pareve,* which are used for foods that are neither meat nor dairy. The Orthodox and Conservative Jews are more likely to observe the laws of *kashrut.* However, many Conservative Jews that follow the laws of *kashrut* in their homes may be less strict when away from their homes.

There are many traditional foods that are often associated with the Sabbath or holidays. For example, chicken soup is commonly served on Friday nights; *matzah,* a piece of unleavened bread resembling a cracker, is eaten during Passover. The foods that are traditionally eaten differ among Jewish groups; for example, the *Sephardim* will eat rice, corn, and peas on Passover while the *Ashkenazim* will not. Specialty foods include hummus (from chickpeas), baba ghanoush (from eggplant), sponge cake (from eggs and flour), and latkas (from potatoes). (See Table 9-1.)

Health and Illness

Providing sensitive and effective perinatal health care for Jewish women and their families involves being knowledgeable of the basic tenets of the religion and the Jewish way of life; this includes their sense of duty to seek and comply with medical advice.[4,10] All practices related to health, illness, sexuality, reproduction, pregnancy, childbirth, and infertility are addressed in the *Halachah.*[7,8,10]

Advances in the evaluation and treatment for infertility present as both blessings and dilemmas to the Orthodox Jewish couple. The ability to more accurately diagnose the cause of infertility and select

Table 9-1
Frequently Eaten Kosher Foods*

Protein	Dairy	Grains	Vegetables	Fruits	Oils	Other
Seafood	Milk	Cereal	Carrots	Dried Fruit	Olive	Nuts
Flounder	Cheese	Kasha	Corn	Apples	Peanut	Seeds
Salmon	Ice Cream	Noodles	Artichokes	Banana	Corn	Honey
(Lox)	Yogurt	Pasta	Zucchini	Cherries	Sesame	Tea
Cod	Butter	Rice	Squash	Peaches		Coffee
Tuna	Eggs	Couscous	Eggplant	Dates		Soda
Whitefish		Bulgur	Olives	Figs		Wine
Snapper		wheat	Potato	Lemon		
Herring			Cucumber	Orange		Sauces
Perch		Breads	Tomato	Pears		Soy
Pike		Challah	Beets	Strawberries		Mustard
		Rye	Onion	Melons		Ketchup
Poultry			Asparagus	Raisins		
Chicken		Flour				
Turkey		Wheat				
		Rye				
Legumes						
Chickpeas						
Lentils						
Beans						

*Orthodox may only eat dairy products and meats under strict supervision.

the most appropriate treatment gives hope to Jewish couples who have been experiencing infertility. However, some of the procedures involved not only challenge the existing Jewish law, but also raise new questions as to their appropriateness in Orthodox Jewish life. Procurement of sperm and invasive procedures and medications that induce a *niddah* state all interfere with sexual relations between the man and woman and, as such, may be viewed as inconsistent with the *Halachah*. Fertility medications and in vitro fertilization, which result in multifetal pregnancy and non-transplanted embryos, present the Jewish couple with difficult decisions to make without clear *Halachah* guidance. In general, homologous artificial insemination and gamete intrafallopian transfers are accepted in Judaism.[11]

Perinatal care for the Orthodox woman and her family must follow the health-related activities that are permitted by the *Torah* and must be consistent with the *Halachah* teachings. However, perinatal care for Conservative or Reform Jewish women and families is similar to the care provided to the general population using Westernized medicine. Despite the different levels of practice, when confronted with life, death, and significant health and illness issues, an individual Jew may vary in his or her observance of the *Torah* and the *Halachah.* As do people of other cultures and religions, Jews will turn to their religious leaders, the rabbis, for guidance in times of stress or when uncertain of how to act.

The health care provider and the observant Jewish perinatal patient and family should collaborate on how to best provide high-quality care while maintaining the sanctity of the Sabbath and holy day observances. If possible, efforts should be made to allow the patient and her visitors uninterrupted prayer time. Although Jewish physicians and nurses are permitted to provide care to patients on the Sabbath and holy days to preserve and protect life and health, a Jew is not permitted to ask another Jew to perform worklike activities on such days. Accordingly, whenever possible, a Jewish health care worker should not be assigned to provide care to an observant Jew on the Sabbath or holy days, except in life-threatening situations. Furthermore, because an Orthodox Jew, and many Conservative Jews, will not use electrical equipment, such as a call light, on the Sabbath and major holy days, the health care professional and ancillary staff should make frequent rounds to check on the status and needs of the perinatal patient and family. A Jew may seek care for minor illnesses on the Sabbath or holy days, but purposely scheduling diagnostic tests and surgery on such days that are not part of emergency care is not permitted.

During fasting periods, Jewish law provides guidance on when and how the perinatal woman fasts so that her health and that of her fetus or breastfeeding baby are not jeopardized. Seriously ill people are mandated to eat and drink. Fasting is never permitted if life will be endangered; however, if modified fasting would not threaten life, then a Jew is obligated to ingest only what is needed to sustain life.

Pregnancy/Prenatal Care

The pregnant Jewish woman is obligated to seek prenatal care and to adhere to health-promoting activities. Prenatal care usually begins in the first trimester. When living in accordance with the *Torah* and *Halachah,* the woman is aware of her menstrual cycles and, thus, alerted to the early signs of pregnancy. Jewish couples practicing all levels of Judaism are receptive to prenatal information about childbirth, newborn care, and breastfeeding.

Orthodox women are more likely to want to seek care from a physician knowledgeable in *Halachah* medical practices. Because a married Jewish woman should avoid being alone with a male who is not her husband, the Orthodox woman may prefer to have a female physician. When a male physician examines a woman, the presence of a female nurse or a female family member is preferred. If necessary, a woman can be in a room with a male physician if the door is unlocked and others are within earshot.[5] During an examination, the woman's body should be fully draped, exposing only the part of the body being assessed, so that modesty is maintained.

The obstetric practice of performing a pelvic examination weekly in the third trimester can be problematic for the observant Jewish woman and her husband. Specifically, if the pelvic examination induces bleeding, the woman is considered to be in a *niddah* state. Accordingly, the pregnant woman and her husband are forbidden to have physical contact until the woman is ritually cleaned in the *mikvah* after the required number of days without bleeding. Many women do not wish to go to a *mikvah* during the latter part of pregnancy and, thus, would rather not be examined internally.[5]

In the more Orthodox communities, grand multiparity and advanced maternal age are common, making them more at risk for related problems, such as placenta previa and Down syndrome. Jewish couples will usually consent to prenatal screening for genetic diseases and fetal abnormalities; this willingness is closely tied to their views concerning termination of pregnancy. Prior to the 40th day after conception, the *Talmud* views the fetus as being made of water, and an abortion may be sanctioned.[10,12] Thus any screening that can foster decisions to be made and acted on before the 40th day after conception are more likely to be accepted by the Orthodox family. Because termination of pregnancy is not acceptable beyond the 40-day limit, alphafetoprotein testing, amniocentesis, and other genetic testing may be rejected,[13] while chorionic villus sampling (CVS) performed as early as 7 weeks' gestation as calculated from the last normal menstrual period or ultrasound may be more appropriate for the Orthodox family.[14] Ultrasounds performed for baseline data and dating of pregnancy are more likely to be accepted by observant Jews.

Several genetic disorders are common among *Ashkenazi* and *Sephardi* Jews. One of the more well-known disorders affecting *Ashkenazi* Jews is Tay-Sachs disease,[15,16] a fatal genetic metabolic disorder of infancy. Because both parents need to be carriers of the trait to have a 25% chance of conceiving a child with the disease, ideally the couple should be tested for the trait before they have children. Because the infant with Tay-Sachs disease will die, many non-*Halachah* practicing Jews seek abortion when the diagnosis has been confirmed by amniocentesis or CVS; when possible, early sampling should be done so that decisions can be made before 40 days after conception. Other genetic disorders that affect *Ashkenazi* Jews include, but are not limited to, Canavan disease,[15,17] Gaucher disease,[15,18] Bloom syndrome,[15] familial dysautonomia,[15,19] Fanconi anemia,[15] Niemann-Pick disease,[15] and cystic fibrosis.[15] *Sephardi* Jewish genetic diseases include familial Mediterranean fever, glucose-6-phosphate dehydrogenase deficiency, and Type III storage disease.[15]

Jewish law dictates that all religious practices be observed, even during pregnancy. However, if a pregnant woman becomes ill, develops a complication, or is physically or emotionally disabled, she is no longer held to the same requirements. For example, a pregnant woman is obligated to fast on Yom Kippur. However, if she experiences preterm labor or illness, she is permitted to drink 45 mL of fluid and eat 30 mL of solid foods in 9 minutes or more. If these rates are not sufficient, then she may repeat that formula or increase the quantity of foods or liquids consumed to the point of restoring and maintaining her own and her fetus's well-being.[10] Foods and liquids high in calories are recommended so that large quantities are not needed. On the fasting days other than Yom Kippur and Tisha B'Av, the pregnant woman is not required to fast but should ingest only enough to ensure her well-being.

Labor and Delivery

From the moment that the membranes rupture, a bloody show appears, or contractions are frequent and so intense that the woman cannot walk without assistance, the pregnant woman is considered to be in labor.[8] On the Sabbath and on holy days, a laboring woman and her husband may travel to the hospital or birthing center, but should not be asked to sign the admission forms and policies.[20] Immediately before or during the Sabbath, labor may be augmented but not induced unless there is a strong medical indication. If the woman is in false labor, it is preferred that she remain at the health care facility until the end of the Sabbath; if this is not possible, then she is permitted to accept a ride home from a non-Jew.

During labor and delivery, the Conservative or Reform husband may be involved with the physical care of his wife by rubbing her back, massaging her body, and wiping her face. The Orthodox husband may touch his wife and provide comfort measures only if she is in early labor and there is no sign of bleeding or ruptured membranes. Once she is considered to be in a *niddah* state, her husband is not permitted to touch her. A female relative or friend often attends the birth and provides physical comfort measures. In addition, the laboring woman frequently engages in prayer as a means of comfort. She may also receive analgesics and anesthetics for control of pain and, if needed, for a cesarean birth. From the time labor begins until 72 hours after birth, the childbearing woman is required to eat and drink, unless medically contraindicated. Even on the fasting days of Yom Kippur and Tisha B'Av, she is encouraged to drink fluids to prevent dehydration. During his wife's labor, an Orthodox husband may remain outside the room reading psalms. However, the woman must be properly draped should he choose to remain in the room; when present, he will usually stand near his wife's head and will avoid looking at the parts of her body that are usually covered.[8] He is not permitted to look at the perineum as his child emerges from the birth canal.

Postpartum and Newborn Care

The postpartum observant Jewish woman prefers to have a female nurse or ancillary health care worker provide physical care. Orthodox women are more likely to feel competent in taking care of their newborns, breastfeeding, and identifying their own needs for rest because they tend to be multiparous and are experienced. In addition, the Orthodox community tends to have large families, and the role of motherhood and activities such as breastfeeding are supported.[4] As such, even first-time Orthodox mothers have had experience taking care of babies and have observed breastfeeding often. Orthodox women experiencing difficulty with breastfeeding are apt to keep it a secret[13]; thus the lactation assistant should discreetly assess and provide related breastfeeding information. The Conservative and Reform Jewish postpartum mother typically does not come from a community where she has had much exposure to raising children and breastfeeding and, thus, is receptive to help and information. Discharge planning and teaching should begin as soon after delivery as possible because an Orthodox woman may ask to be released early because of the Sabbath.[13]

The care of the hospitalized postpartum woman who is an Orthodox Jew must be modified on the Sabbath and on Jewish holy days. She cannot tear paper or spread ointment, or use a washcloth, sponge, or soap bar on the Sabbath and holy days.[9,10] The health care provider can accommodate these taboos by opening the outer packaging of self-care items such as tissues and peri-pads, providing liquid soap in a bottle that can be sprayed over the area to be cleaned, and providing nonabsorbent gauze with ointment already placed on it. When bathing the new mother, a gloved hand should be used and the use of a sponge or cloth should be avoided.[10] Providers should also use liquid soap when washing their own hands prior to taking care of the patient.

The *Halachah* guides breastfeeding and breast care. On the Sabbath, for example, the mother may only express milk when severely engorged or when it will benefit the baby, such as when breast milk needs to be brought to the hospital for an ill infant; however, milk that is expressed for her comfort is discarded.[10] Also, she may only use nonabsorbent gauze to cleanse her nipples.[10]

Jewish family members tend to be very involved in the care of the postpartum mother and her newborn. Grandparents and other relatives visit the mother and new baby, and often are available to help care for other children at home while the woman is in the hospital or at home. Husbands who are Conservative or Reform Jews tend to provide support and care to their wives and the newborn.

According to Jewish law, the postpartum woman is in the *niddah* state and the couple cannot touch each other until after the ritual bath. Still, the husband is supportive of his wife and does interact with his newborn. According to the *Halachah,* a woman may go to the *mikvah* 7 days after the birth of a son and 14 days after the birth of a daughter, provided she has had 7 days without bleeding.[7,8] However, these rules are rarely applicable because most postpartum women have a bloody vaginal discharge longer than 7 days after delivery. After a miscarriage or abortion, if the gender of the baby has not been determined, the woman is required to wait at least 14 days before going to the *mikvah,* provided that 7 days have been without bleeding.

The woman who observes the laws of *kashrut* continues to do so postpartum. A kosher diet should be ordered. She may wish to have food brought in from home to supplement her diet. Some facilities provide a separate refrigerator for the Orthodox to store their food. In addition, the observant woman should be provided with a basin, a cup, and a water pitcher to wash her hands before every meal.[9,13]

Halachah law does permit the woman who is less that 30 days postpartum and/or lactating to forego the customary 6-hour wait between eating meat and dairy, and allows her to eat dairy within 1 hour of meat.[10] According to Jewish law, fasting is not permitted for the first 3 days postpartum and is not mandatory for the next 4 days.[9,10] A mother who is breastfeeding may fast as long as it does not interfere with lactation. When infants are fed formula, the bottles must be prepared prior to the Sabbath and then warmed by placing the bottle in a bowl containing hot water obtained from a pot that has been left on a fire for this purpose.

The care of the newborn on weekdays and non-holy days is routine care. There is no prescribed cord care. However, on the Sabbath and Jewish holy days, a cotton ball or paper tissue with light petrolatum oil can be used to cleanse the newborn diaper area because washing with a sponge or washcloth and using a bar of soap are prohibited.[8] If absolutely needed, the diaper area may be sprayed with a liquid soap solution from a plastic bottle.[8] Ointments are also not permitted on the Sabbath or holy days; thus when petroleum jelly needs to be applied to the circumcised penis or diaper area, it should be applied to a gauze pad before the Sabbath.[10] Because diapers may not be flushed or rinsed on the Sabbath or holy days,[8] disposable diapers are often preferred for these days. If cloth diapers are used and become soiled, they are placed in a closed container without any treatments until after the end of the Sabbath or holy day.

The Jewish male newborn is circumcised on the eighth day after birth as a sign of the covenant with God. Although the ritual circumcision is called *brit milah* in Hebrew, in the United States, the term *bris* is commonly used for the religious circumcision. The *brit milah* is performed by a *mohel*, a learned and religious Jew who is trained in both the surgical procedure and the special prayers.[2] Similar to nonritual circumcisions, the *mohel* will apply gauze with petroleum jelly to the penis immediately after the circumcision is performed, and the parents may be instructed to apply an antibacterial ointment for a day or 2.

To attend a *brit* is a blessing; thus many family members and friends are invited. After the circumcision, a blessing is said over wine and the baby is named. The ceremony ends with the guests singing and wishing good fortune and luck. This is followed by a celebration.

Healthy male infants undergo the *brit* on the eighth day of life, even if it is the Sabbath or Yom Kippur.[2] However, a *brit* cannot be performed on the Sabbath or a holy day if the baby was delivered by cesarean section or if the *brit* was delayed because of medical reasons. An infant with a localized illness or injury may be circumcised as soon as recovery is evident. The infant with physiologic jaundice may not be circumcised until his color is normal. An infant with a cleft lip or palate can be circumcised if otherwise healthy. The presence of the following conditions prohibit circumcision on the eighth day: fever of 38°C or higher; pathologic, multisystem illness; anemia; unresolved physiologic jaundice; incubator required for care; history of 2 brothers that died from circumcision; and the death of a twin within 8 days of the birth.[10] A *brit* and baby naming may occur in the hospital when the mother or baby has been ill. The family may require a private room in which the ceremony and celebration may take place.[20]

Traditionally, Jewish male infants are named on the eighth day at the *brit*, and female infants are named in the synagogue on the first Sabbath after the birth or soon thereafter. Some Reform families will have a naming ceremony at home for their female infant. Many Orthodox Jews will not tell anyone the name of the infant until the naming ceremony[13]; thus the birth record may be incomplete at the time the newborn is discharged from the hospital or birthing center.

In the United States, it is customary for Jewish male and female infants to be given a Hebrew and a secular name. A Hebrew name is required for men when called on to read from the *Torah* and also for any Jewish contract.[2,9] *Ashkenazim* tend to name their infants after deceased relatives, believing that if an infant is named after the living, the angel of death might get confused and by mistake take the child instead of the elder.[3] *Sephardim* traditionally name their children after the living, believing that the angel of death would err on the side of longevity.[2] Jews from Balkan nations such as Greece often name their firstborn male *bechor* and female *bechora,* meaning "oldest."[9]

According to the *Torah,* when the firstborn to a woman is delivered vaginally and is a son, he belongs to God. He can be freed from the obligation of dedicating his life to God's service through a ceremony called *Pidyon Ha-ben,* conducted at home on the 31st day of life. If the firstborn was delivered by cesarean section or the mother had a previous pregnancy that resulted in miscarriage or abortion after the 40th day of gestation, the ceremony is not conducted.[9] Additionally, a firstborn son whose mother or father is a descendant of the ancient Hebrew tribes of *Kohen* or *Levites* cannot be released from his obligation to priesthood. Reform Jews do not believe that priesthood is inherited.

Family Planning

Although conservative and Reform Jewish couples are more likely to use some form of contraception during their married life, most Orthodox Jewish couples consider contraception to be in conflict with the first commandment to procreate. However the commandment to procreate is an obligation of the male and not the female, thus the use of contraceptives when medically indicated is permitted.[4] Of the contraceptive methods, hormonal interventions and birth control pills are probably the most compatible with Judaic beliefs; however, because they are not free of harmful side effects and may induce breakthrough bleeding, they may be rejected.[6] The rhythm method is not acceptable because it would necessitate almost total abstinence when combined with the laws of *niddah*.[5] Vasectomies, tubal ligation, and male condoms are also unacceptable to the Orthodox.

Bioethical Dilemmas

The role of Jewish theology in bioethics is not new. Throughout Judaic history, Jewish leaders have responded to the challenges posed by advancements in medicine and technology, as well as changes in public law that influence health care practices. Answers to bioethical questions may, in part, be addressed in the *Torah,* the *Talmud,* and the written *Halachah.* However, bioethical issues that are not sufficiently addressed in previous written Jewish law become the focus of modern day discussions among rabbinical authorities. The current written opinions of the rabbinical authorities are found in a body of publications termed *Responsa*.[6] Drawing on the *Responsa,* other rabbis provide guidance to Jewish individuals, families, and communities faced with making bioethical decisions.

Death/Burial Rites

When there is a perinatal loss, whether by miscarriage, stillbirth, or neonatal death, the foundation of the Jewish home is shaken and the husband and wife, individually and as a couple, are affected. Most practicing Jewish couples, and many of those who have an ethnic but non-religious affiliation, will seek the advice and comfort offered by a rabbi when faced with a loss late in pregnancy or after birth. Similar to other couples experiencing a perinatal loss, the Jewish couple wants to know what caused the loss of their baby. Although autopsies are usually not permitted, a rabbi may sanction the procedure if it will provide information that might help to prevent a future perinatal loss.[10,21] If an autopsy is performed, the remains are buried according to Jewish law.

Jewish law provides guidance as to how one conducts oneself when confronted with perinatal loss. Special death rituals and prayers help the Jewish couple cope with the loss, receive comfort, and sustain hope.[21] A fetus of less than 5 months' gestation is not considered viable and, thus, burial and mourning rituals do not apply. A fetus of 5 gestational months or greater, a stillborn, or an infant that dies after birth are buried on the sacred grounds of a Jewish cemetery.[21] Jewish funerals are held as soon as possible, usually within 24 hours excluding the Sabbath. In situations where the mother is still recovering from the birth, the funeral may be delayed until she is able to attend.[21]

A modified graveside funeral, with only a rabbi and the immediate family present, is often conducted for a stillborn or a baby that died soon after birth.[21] Following the burial, the parents may observe a 24-hour *shiva*, a period of mourning during which friends and family visit the home and provide help.

The rituals prescribed in Jewish law differ for infants born alive and those that were stillborn. All deceased infants who had been born alive receive the ritual washing called *taharah*.[21] Newborns who live less than 8 days may be circumcised[21,22] and named at the burial. An infant that dies after 30 days of life is given a funeral, and the family will observe the traditional mourning rituals. These rituals include performing *keria*, sitting *shiva*, and reciting *Kaddish*. *Keria* is the rending or tearing of a garment as an expression of one's grief over the death of a family member.[9] Reform and Conservative Jews often wear a black ribbon that is cut, instead of tearing an actual article of clothing. The garment or ribbon is worn the entire week after the funeral during the *shiva* period. *Keria* is not performed when an infant has not lived for 30 days.[9] When the newborn lives for at least 30 days, the *shiva* lasts 3 to 7 days. During the *shiva*, the observant Jew will light a memorial candle, cover mirrors, sit in low chairs, refrain from wearing leather shoes, and not work or engage in business. After the *shiva,* some parents may choose to go to the synagogue daily for 1 month to recite *Kaddish.* On the anniversary of the neonatal death, or stillborn, the family may observe *Yahreit,* as evidenced by lighting a candle, reciting a prayer, and making a donation.[23]

When a child is born with mental disabilities, parental concern for the child's future is universal. Jewish parents may have additional cultural challenges to overcome. The *Torah* views all humans as created in God's image; thus the competent and mentally challenged individuals are valued.[24] Furthermore, Jewish law encourages Jews to take care of the less fortunate and provides the opportunity for Jews to live together side by side. Anecdotal reports of mentally disabled children participating in rites of passage (eg, having a *Bar Mitzvah*[25]) and the support by rabbinical leaders for group homes for the mentally disabled as a requirement of the *halachah*[24] serve as examples as to how to ensure that the mentally disabled Jew is embraced into the Jewish community.

Termination of pregnancy is never taken lightly by observant Jewish couples. They will usually consult with a rabbi when making a decision of this magnitude. Because prior to the 40th day after conception the fetus is viewed as being made of water, an abortion may be sanctioned.[10,11] Abortion may be performed in certain situations beyond the 40th day after conception.[10,11,26] If the mother's life is physically or emotionally endangered, the fetus is viewed as an aggressor and the pregnancy may be terminated.[27] If the fetus is anencephalic, an abortion is sanctioned.[10] When other fetal anomalies or genetic diseases are diagnosed during the pregnancy, a rabbi should be consulted to determine whether an abortion is permissible. In a multiple pregnancy when there is little hope for all the fetuses to survive, it is difficult to say which fetus is the aggressor. Multifetal reduction may be acceptable from the point that it is performed to prevent complications and premature birth that are due to multifetal gestation.[6,26] When multifetal reduction is performed, selection should be randomly determined and not based on gender or the presence of a non–life-threatening deformity.[28]

More recently, in vitro fertilization has raised the issue of how to dispose of non-transplanted eggs. Because some authorities view a non-transplanted embryo as not a potential fetus, it may be discarded; but all do not hold this view.[6,29,30] The controversial technological advances in stem cell research have further complicated the issue.[30]

Every Jewish Woman Is Unique

Providing care to Jewish perinatal patients requires that the health care professional and ancillary health care workers assess and acknowledge the degree to which the Jewish laws are practiced by the patient and her family. A willingness to understand and respect the religious and ethnic practices of the patient and her family is essential for establishing a therapeutic relationship.

Perinatal Health Care Issues of Jewish Women: Key Highlights

Demographic/Psychosocial/Spiritual Characteristics

- Jews live in all parts of the world and speak a variety of languages; although Hebrew is the official language of Judaism, Yiddish is a common dialect that is based on German.
- Because the history of the Jewish people is so tied in with religious persecution and exile from their homelands, affiliation and kinship with other Jews is important.
- The feeling of kinship felt by Jewish people of varying nationalities is partly perpetuated through their common religious and cultural practices.
- The Jewish law commands Jews to be fertile and increase in number.
- Jews are duty-bound to seek and comply with medical advice.

- The Jewish people believe in one spiritual, moral, and ethical God.
- The *Torah* is the Jewish Bible; the *Talmud* is a collection of laws.
- The *Halachah* is a collection of rabbinical decisions that apply Jewish law to daily situations.
- There are 3 levels of practicing Judaism: Orthodox, Conservative, and Reform. Individuals vary in their practice; the Orthodox tend to be the most observant Jews.
- Prayer is an essential component of daily life for observant Jews.
- The Jewish Sabbath starts Friday at sundown and ends Saturday at sundown.
- On the Sabbath and the holy days, the Orthodox refrain from work-related activities such as operating electrical appliances, riding in a car or elevator, turning on lights, striking a match, writing, and tearing paper.
- Fasting is observed on major holy days; on Yom Kippur, they cannot eat for 25 hours after sundown.
- Fasting is prohibited during illness or if it could harm a fetus or breastfeeding infant.
- A Jew cannot ask another Jew to do work on the Sabbath or a holy day.
- Jewish physicians and nurses may provide care to protect life.
- A Jew should not schedule routine diagnostic tests on Sabbath or holy days.
- The marriage bond is deemed an opportunity for holiness.
- Intimacy and love are important; sexual intercourse is for pleasure and procreation.
- The laws of *niddah* are a set of rules and rituals that focus on restrictions in the wife's sexual availability.
- The wife is considered impure when menstruating or experiencing uterine bleeding.
- A ritual bath, called *mikvah*, restores purity.

- Orthodox women cannot unduly expose their bodies; they must wear wigs or other head coverings.
- Meat and dairy products cannot be eaten at the same time, and separate dishes, pots, pans, and utensils are needed for each; *pareve* is neither meat nor dairy, it is neutral.

Prenatal Care

- Homologous artificial insemination and gamete intrafallopian transfer may be acceptable methods for overcoming infertility.
- Jewish women are obligated to seek care during pregnancy.
- The Orthodox are more likely to seek a doctor who is knowledgeable in *Halachah* medical practices.
- Orthodox women should not be alone with a man who is not her husband; a female should be present in the examination room.
- Unless necessary, pelvic examinations should be avoided because they may induce a *niddah* state, and women may prefer to avoid the ritual bath during pregnancy.
- Grand multiparity and advanced maternal age are common among Orthodox women.
- During pregnancy, Orthodox women observe all religious practices unless ill.

Prenatal Testing

- Conservative and Reform Jews usually accept genetic testing and screening for abnormalities; Orthodox women may be less willing due to their beliefs in procreation.
- *Ashkenazi* Jews are at risk for Tay-Sachs disease.

Pregnancy Diet

- Pregnant women must fast on Yom Kippur, but they can modify the fast to avoid dehydration.
- During pregnancy, food or liquid should be taken when hungry, ill, in preterm labor, or if conceived in vitro; if needed, they should consume high-calorie foods and observe a modified fast.

Labor and Delivery

- An Orthodox patient or family should not be asked to sign admission forms on the Sabbath or Jewish holy days.
- The laboring woman may ride in a car on the Sabbath.
- Induction of labor on the Sabbath should be avoided; augmentation of labor is permitted.
- An Orthodox woman is considered *niddah* when she has intense contractions, a bloody show, or a dilated cervix.
- It is very important to drape the woman's private parts at all times.
- The laboring woman should not fast.
- Analgesia and anesthesia are permissible.

Postpartum Care

- A female nurse is preferred.
- On the Sabbath, a postpartum mother cannot use a washcloth, sponge, or bar of soap; nor can she spread ointment.

Postpartum Diet

- The Orthodox woman must observe the laws of *kashrut* during the postpartal period.
- Hands must be washed before every meal.
- Fasting should not be observed for the first 3 days after birth and is non-mandatory for the next 4 days.

Neonatal Care

- Orthodox women are usually competent with newborns due to prior experience.
- There is no prescribed cord care.
- On the Sabbath, a plastic spray bottle with liquid soap is needed; the Orthodox cannot use a washcloth or rinse out diapers.
- On the eighth day, a ritual circumcision *(brit milah* or *bris)* is performed by a *mohel.*
- Circumcision cannot be done if the infant is ill, has jaundice, needs an incubator, or is febrile, or if there is a history of sibling death from the procedure.

- Males are named on the eighth day of life, females on the first Sabbath after birth.
- *Ashkenazim* name the baby after deceased relatives; *Sephardim* name after the living.
- If discharge of the mother or baby is delayed, the *brit* and naming may be done in the hospital.
- A *Pidyon Ha-Ben* ceremony is performed on the 31st day to free a firstborn son from dedicating his life to God's service.

Breastfeeding/Breast Care
- An Orthodox woman may not admit she is having trouble with breastfeeding.
- On the Sabbath, Orthodox women cannot use absorbent cotton to cleanse their nipples.
- Breast milk can only be expressed on the Sabbath if needed by a hospitalized baby.

Family Planning
- Contraception is more acceptable to Reform and Conservative Jews than to Orthodox couples.
- Hormonal interventions such as the birth control pill may be acceptable to some Orthodox women.
- Vasectomies, tubal ligations, and condom use are not acceptable practices to the Orthodox.

Family Involvement
- Often, a female relative or friend will be with the Orthodox woman during labor; the husband either stays outside or at the head of the bed. The family is very involved during pregnancy and after birth.
- An Orthodox husband cannot touch his wife whenever she is in a *niddah* state, a minimum of 7 to 14 days after giving birth.
- Conservative and Reform husbands tend to be involved with helping their wives before, during, and after birth in the care of their newborns.

Pregnancy Termination/Miscarriage

- Perinatal loss and abortion is more acceptable before the 40th day after conception because the Orthodox believe that a fetus is made of water until that time; after the 40th day, abortion may be done if the mother's life is endangered and a rabbi sanctions it.
- Although it is a relatively new theological issue, multifetal reduction may be acceptable.

Bioethical Dilemmas

- Bioethical issues may, in part, be addressed in the *Torah,* the *Talmud,* and the written *Halachah.*
- Bioethical issues not sufficiently addressed in previous written Jewish law are discussed among rabbinical authorities and published in a body of publications termed *Responsa.* Guidance to Jewish individuals, families, and communities faced with making bioethical decisions are based on the *Responsa.*

Death/Burial Rites

- Judaism celebrates life and procreation; perinatal death is a family tragedy.
- A deceased fetus is buried in a cemetery if it died after the fifth month of gestation.
- The rituals of mourning and burial are modified for stillborns and infants who die soon after birth.
- Burial must take place within 24 hours unless the mother needs to recover from delivery.
- Mourners of an infant who lives 30 days tear an article of clothing or wear torn ribbon *(keria),* sit *shiva* for 7 days, and say a mourner's prayer for 30 days after the *shiva.*

References

1. Donin HH. *To Be a Jew*. New York, NY: Basic Books; 1972
2. Diamant A. *The New Jewish Baby Book*. Woodstock, VT: Jewish Lights Publishing; 2001
3. Sternberg R. *The Sephardic Kitchen*. New York, NY: HarperCollins Publishers; 1996
4. Schenker JG. Women's reproductive health: monotheistic religious perspectives. *Int J Gynecol Obstet*. 2000;70:77–86
5. Feldman P. Sexuality, birth control and childbirth in orthodox Jewish tradition. *Can Med Assoc J*. 1992;146:29–33
6. Grazi RV, Wolowelsky JB. Multifetal pregnancy reduction and disposal of untransplanted embryos in contemporary Jewish law and ethics. *Am J Obstet Gynecol*. 1991;165:1268–1271
7. Abramov T, Touger M. *The Secret of Jewish Femininity*. Southfield, MI: Targum Press; 1988
8. Tendler MD. *Pardes Rimonim. A Manual for the Jewish Family*. Hoboken, NJ: KTAV Publishing House; 1988
9. Kolatch AJ. *The Jewish Home Advisor*. Middle Village, NY: Jonathan David Publishers; 1998
10. Abraham AS. *The Comprehensive Guide to Medical Halachah*. Jerusalem, Israel: Feldheim Publishers; 1996
11. Hirsh JF, Bhagwati SN, Epstein F, Hoppe-Hirsch E, Mutluer S, Raimondi AJ. Medical abortion: ethics, laws and religious points of view. *Childs Nerv Syst*. 1996;12:507–514
12. Waterhouse C. Midwifery for orthodox Jewish women. *Modern Midwif*. 1994;4:11–14
13. Lutwak RA, Ney AM, White JE. Maternity nursing and Jewish law. *Maternal Child Nurs*. 1988;13:44–88
14. Wapner RJ, Evans MI, Davis G, et al. Procedural risks versus theology: Chorionic villus sampling for Orthodox Jews at less than 8 weeks' gestation. *Am J Obstet Gynecol*. 2002;186:1133–1136
15. Center for Jewish Genetic Disorders, Children's Memorial Hospital *Jewish Genetic Disorders*. Available at: http://www.jewishgenetics.org/gendis.htm. Accessed February 15, 2003
16. Kaback MM. Hexosaminidase A deficiency. In: *Gene Reviews*. Seattle, WA: University of Washington; 2001. Available at: http://www.geneclinics.org. Accessed February 15, 2003
17. Matalon R. Canavan disease. In: *Gene Reviews*. Seattle, WA: University of Washington; 2001

18. Pastores GM. Gaucher disease. In: *Gene Reviews.* Seattle, WA: University of Washington; 2000. Available at: http://www.geneclinics.org. Accessed February 15, 2003

19. Shohat M. Familial dysautonomia. In: *Gene Reviews.* Seattle, WA: University of Washington; 2003. Available at: http://www.geneclinics.org. Accessed February 15, 2003

20. De Sevo MR. Keeping the faith. *Lifelines.* August 1997:46–49

21. Cardin NB. *Tears of Sorrow, Seeds of Hope.* Woodstock, VT: Jewish Lights Publishing; 1999

22. Kolatch AJ. *The Jewish Mourner's Book of Why.* Middle Village, NY: Jonathan David Publishers; 1993

23. Dickstein S. Confronting stillbirth: Jewish ritual and halakhah: a responsum from the conservative movement's Committee on Jewish Law and Standards. *JTS Magazine.* 2000;9(2). Available at: http://www.jtsa.edu/news/jtsmag/9.2/hatesh.shtml. Accessed February 15, 2003

24. Rosen JS. Caring for our kinsmen: a responsum from the Committee on Jewish Law and Standards. *JTS Magazine.* 2001;10(2). Available at: http://www.jtsa.edu/news/jtsmag/10.2/hateshuvah.shtml. Accessed February 15, 2003

25. Schwartz PR. Into the covenant. *JTS Magazine.* 1999;8(3). Available at: http://www.jtsa.edu/news/jtsmag/8.3/itc.shtml. Accessed February 15, 2003

26. Grazi RV. *Be Fruitful and Multiply.* Ma'ale Amos, Israel: Genesis Jerusalem Press; 1994

27. Eisenberg D. Abortion and halacha. *Jewish Virtual Library.* Available at: http://www.us-israel.org/jsource/Judaism/abortion.html. Accessed February 15, 2003

28. Chertok I. Multifetal pregnancy reduction and halakha. *Early Pregnancy Biol Med.* 2001;5:201–210. Available at: http://www.earlypregnancy.org). Accessed February 15, 2003

29. Grazi RV, Wolowelsky JB. Homologous artificial insemination (AIH) and gamete intrafallopian transfer (GIFT) in Roman Catholicism and Halachic Judaism. *Int Fertility.* 1993;38:75–78

30. Eisenberg D. Stem cell research in Jewish law. *Jewish Law.* 2001. Available at: http://www.jlaw.com/Articles/stemcellres.html. Accessed February 15, 2003

10
Perinatal Health Care Issues
of Korean Women

Luella Steil

Korea has one of the highest population densities in the world, estimated to be 459 people per square kilometer (1,188 per square mile).[1] As a result, Koreans have learned to cope with crowded conditions and live in harmony with one another. From an early age, they are taught to value the group's priority over individual desires and needs. Politeness is very important and extends to generosity in gift giving, food preparation for guests, and financial transactions.[2] The literacy rate among Koreans is estimated at 93%.[2] The political divisions between the north and south of Korea have created deep tensions between the 2 communities.

Although Korea has its own unique culture, the Chinese influence is strong, dating as far back as 108 BC,[1] and has been enriched by the historic traditions of Confucianism and Buddhism. In recent years, modernization, urbanization, and Westernization have weakened these influences. Traditional beliefs regarding the role of women in society, however, are adhered to more so than those that influence other aspects of Korean life.[2] For example, illegitimacy is socially and culturally unacceptable and will lead to either marriage or an elective abortion. In addition, obedience to the males and elders of the family is still prevalent.[2] Nevertheless, when a Korean woman seems unopinionated or behaves in a quiet, passive, docile manner, "yes" usually means, "I heard you" not "I will do it."[2]

Korean immigration to the United States began around 1904. It increased greatly after the passage of the Immigration and Naturalization Act of 1965. By 1988, 1.2 million of the 2 million Koreans living abroad resided in the United States.[2,3] Approximately 95% of Korean immigrants have settled in urban areas throughout the 50 states. Most of the immigrant population is of childbearing age,[3] making it likely that, at some time or other, a perinatal health care worker will provide care for a Korean client.

Health and Illness

Most Koreans believe in a traditional view of health that has been mainly influenced by Chinese culture. This view believes in opposing and uniting forces, the Um (Yin in Chinese) and the Yang, and also believes in the presence of 5 elements of the universe (earth, water, fire, metal, and wood), all of which must be in harmony. Disease results when there is an imbalance of any of these components. Health exists when there is balance in one's universe and no disturbance in the Um and the Yang.[2] Traditional Koreans have a great respect for people in authority, including the health care worker.

Koreans living in the United States may use both the American medical system and traditional Korean medicine. Korean physicians adapt their treatments accordingly; however, it is important for the American health care worker to be aware of this because of the danger of harmful chemical interactions.

Pregnancy/Prenatal Care

In Korea, the rate of maternal deaths due to pregnancy, delivery, and puerperal complications was 2.0 per 10,000 live births in 1996.[3] In 1993 the infant mortality rate was 9.9 per 1,000 live births. The low birth weight rate was 6.0 to 6.4, and the death rate for complications of low birth weight was 41.8.[4] In Korea, pregnancy is considered a family affair and a normal developmental process, not a pathologic process that necessitates the use of high-tech medicine (see Interview).

Some feel that childbearing itself can restore an imbalanced body. A common belief among Korean women is that *tae mong*, a dream of conception, occurs prior to conceiving. Dreams about snakes and other animals are thought to predict a boy while fruits, flowers, and small objects are thought to predict a girl. Once a woman has had a *tae mong,* she begins the practice of *tae kyo,* which is a set of rules and taboos to be followed for achieving a safe childbirth.[5] *Tae kyo* promotes the physical and mental well-being of the mother and protects the fetus. The whole family participates in making sure that the pregnant woman is encouraged to read classical literature and view beautiful art objects; maintain a serene, optimistic attitude; think about pretty things; and have only happy thoughts. There are many taboos Korean women observe during pregnancy. For example, they should avoid handling unclean things and killing any living creature; stealing or doing mischievous things; consuming such foods as duck, chicken, fish without scales, squid, and crab, because the unborn child might resemble them; eating rabbit, because it could cause a transverse presentation; and writing one's name in red, because it could bring bad luck.[2,5] In addition, a *shaman* may be used to exorcise evil spirits from the body.[2]

Although no specific diet is prescribed during pregnancy, Koreans tend to have a high incidence of lactose intolerance, making them prone to avoid dairy products.[6] Eggs are eaten by some Koreans and not accepted by others. Rice is included at every meal. Because many of the foods that are avoided are proteins, there is a potential for the mother to consume a diet that is less than adequate for maintaining a healthy pregnancy.

Koreans believe in delivering a small infant, then helping it to grow big. Thus some women will wear an abdominal binder beginning at 20 weeks' gestation, while others will work very hard during the second half of pregnancy, believing that this will help to ensure a small baby.[2]

Korean women usually begin prenatal care around the fifth month of pregnancy, waiting to be certain that they are pregnant prior to seeking care. A female health care provider is generally preferred. In traditional Korean medicine, diagnosis is made through history-taking, visual observation, and quality of pulses. Thus many Korean women expect to receive care without a physical examination; in fact, some may never have had a Pap smear.[2] The American health care worker needs to be aware of this and sensitive to the Korean woman's need for modesty.

Labor and Delivery

In Korea, a midwife, who was a woman of middle age with many sons and much experience delivering babies,[5] traditionally attended women in birth. Her role was that of a mental guide during labor rather than an obstetric care provider.[2] Men were not allowed in the room of confinement until after the placenta was burned, buried, or submerged in the ocean. Childless women were also excluded, for it was feared they would bring misfortune to the baby.[5]

Today most births take place in the hospital, and husbands do not usually participate during the birth experience. Koreans tend to prefer an unmedicated, natural childbirth. The laboring woman is allowed to walk, squat, or crawl as she wishes, but stoic endurance of pain is encouraged. In Korea, the placenta is usually buried, burned, or put into the ocean.

Postpartum and Newborn Care

The focus of postpartum care in Korea is allowing the new mother to rest and be with her newborn. Bed rest may range from 7 days to 3 months; however, the average is 21 days. It is believed that exposure to cold during the postpartum period will cause chronic illnesses such as arthritis.[2] Thus the environment of the new mother is kept warm and free of cold drafts, and the newborn must be kept swaddled. Seaweed soup (see recipe) and steamed rice are considered essentials for the new mother. A soft diet is also required to allow the teeth to recover from pregnancy, and all food and drink must be warm.

The mother-in-law or other female relatives will stay with the new mother for the first month, performing household chores and allowing her to focus on herself and her newborn. People who are in mourning are not permitted to visit, as this would interfere with the newborn's health and the mother's recovery.[2]

The rate of breastfeeding in Korea decreased from 50% in 1985 to 11.4% in 1991, with an insufficient milk supply (42.5%) and the baby's preference for cow milk (17.5%) cited by mothers as the main reasons for not nursing their babies.[7] Those who do breastfeed often differ as to when it should be initiated. Some believe it should begin at birth while others think it should not be started until the third day after birth. Infants are breastfed on demand for as long as 2 years. If engorgement occurs, the breasts are massaged. Infant feeding choice has been found to be the one area where an Americanized Korean mother is most likely to deviate from her traditional teachings and choose bottle-feeding.[5]

Newborns are not allowed to cry for any length of time and frequently sleep with their mothers. The family usually waits for more than a month before taking the infant out into public.[5] Although fathers tend to have minimal involvement in the care of the newborn, this is changing. Sons tend to be more highly valued than daughters are; nevertheless, all infants are welcomed and indulged. Infant vaccination is a high priority for the Korean government, and the rate of vaccination in 1991 was reported at 95.8%.[7]

Family Planning

Although the Korean government has encouraged contraception since the early 1960s, there are no governmental programs that officially control or promote family planning; still, the rate of contraception was estimated to be 80.5% in 1991.[8] Although the emphasis on producing a male child to care for parents in their old age is diminishing in Korea, the more modern and educated woman may continue to bear children until she has a son.[2] Coitus interruptus or douching after intercourse are prevalent contraceptive practices among Korean women. Elective abortion may also be used as a fertility control method.[2]

Death/Burial Rites

When a Korean dies, his or her name is crossed out or written in red ink.[2] In addition, Koreans tend to view a stillbirth as a baby that was never born. Generally, the hospital disposes of the stillborn and no funeral rites are observed.

Every Korean Woman Is Unique

Just as every woman born in America may feel different about pregnancy, birth, and parenting, so does every Korean woman. The information presented in this chapter is meant to provide general guidelines for caring for Korean women during the perinatal period. The reader is cautioned to carefully assess the cultural, religious, and health beliefs of every woman in their care.

Korean culture has a strong influence on the childbearing Korean family. This influence can be summarized by the following 4 points: (1) Koreans view health and pregnancy holistically; (2) Koreans are influenced by Eastern and Western views, although the degree of influence will vary among individuals; (3) the expectant Korean mother may need to be provided with scientific health information; and (4) pregnancy is a developmental and familial task.[2]

Perinatal Health Care Issues of Korean Women: Key Highlights

Psychosocial/Spiritual Characteristics

- Politeness, docility, quietness, obedience to the males and elders of the family, and seeking group approval are common traits.
- Korean women may seem unopinionated; however, "yes" may mean "I heard you" not "I will do it."
- A shaman may be used to exorcise evil spirits from the body.

Prenatal Care

- Prenatal care is usually started around the fifth month of pregnancy.
- Korean women may have never had a Pap smear previously and expect to have their modesty respected during physical examinations; they tend to prefer female health care providers.
- A combination of American biomedical and Korean traditional medicine may be used in treating physical ailments, creating a risk of harmful chemical interactions.
- To keep the fetus small, some may work very hard during the second half of pregnancy and wear an abdominal binder after the 20th week of gestation.

Prenatal Testing

- Pregnancy is considered a normal developmental process, not a pathologic process that necessitates the use of high-tech medicine.

Pregnancy Diet

- No specific diet is prescribed during pregnancy. Rice is included at every meal (occasionally noodles are substituted for rice).
- Korean pregnant women are to think about pretty things and to have happy thoughts.
- Koreans have a high incidence of lactose intolerance and, thus, may avoid dairy products; many do not eat eggs.
- Eating rabbit is thought to cause a transverse presentation while duck, chicken, fish without scales, squid, and crab are avoided so that the child will not resemble these foods.
- The Korean diet during pregnancy may be less than adequate in protein.

Pregnancy-Related Beliefs/Taboos

- It is believed that pregnant women should not steal, do mischievous things, handle unclean things, or kill any living creature.
- Writing their names in red is thought to bring bad luck.

Labor and Delivery

- Unmedicated, natural childbirth is preferred, and stoic endurance of pain during labor is encouraged.
- It is acceptable for women to walk, squat, or crawl in labor.
- The placenta is buried, burned, or put into the ocean.
- Today most births are in hospitals; husbands do not generally participate in the birth experience.

Postpartum Care

- New mothers are encouraged to maintain bed rest with bed baths for an average of 21 days.
- Cold winds and cold water are believed to trigger arthritis/chronic illness and, thus, are to be avoided.

Postpartum Diet

- Seaweed soup (see recipe) and steamed rice are considered essential components of the daily diet.
- Cold drinks or foods are to be avoided.
- A soft diet is followed to allow the teeth to recover from pregnancy.

Neonatal Care

- Newborns are kept swaddled to avoid exposure to cold draft.
- Infants are not allowed to cry for any length of time and may sleep with the mother.
- An infant should be older than 1 month before going out into public places.

Breastfeeding/Breast Care

- Most Korean women choose to bottle-feed.
- Breastfeeding on demand is usually promoted for up to 2 years.
- Seaweed soup (see recipe) is eaten for 1 month postpartum to ensure good milk production.
- If engorgement occurs, husbands may be taught to massage the breasts.

- In severe cases of engorgement, cooked bean sprouts may be wrapped in a towel and laid over the breasts.

Family Planning

- Inaccurate contraceptive information is common.
- Ineffective birth control practices, such as coitus interruptus or douching after intercourse, are still prevalent among some Korean women.

Family Involvement

- A female stays with the new mother for the first month, performing household chores and permitting the mother to care for her baby.

Pregnancy Termination/Miscarriage

- Elective abortions are common, especially in cases of illegitimate pregnancy.

Death/Burial Rites

- After a person dies, their name is crossed out or written in red ink.
- A stillbirth is viewed as a baby that was never born; no funeral rites are observed and hospital disposal is preferred.

Interview With a Korean Immigrant

This author had the privilege of interviewing a Korean immigrant about her beliefs related to pregnancy and childbirth. Younghee (a pseudonym) is active in Korean organizations and attends Korean postpartum women in the state of Georgia. The interviews took place in 1997 and again in 1999. During the exchange of information, it was quite evident that many of her beliefs were steeped in Korean tradition.

Younghee adheres to the ideas of tae kyo. "When I was pregnant, I was supposed to think pleasant thoughts. I was to choose food by how it looks, for example I was to choose the prettiest apple." She related that she was taught in the middle-school grades that childbirth was a natural process that could be endured without the use of drugs. She was also taught that breastfeeding was best. Younghee adhered to the concept of a warm environment during the postpartum period. She not only recommended warm food and drink, she also stated that it should be soft to allow her teeth to heal from the pregnancy. Thus she reflected a holistic view of pregnancy. Younghee believed in the use of rice in the daily diet, before and after the birth. She stated that some women will develop an intolerance to rice during pregnancy and will switch to eating noodles. She talked about the importance of seaweed soup (see recipe) postpartum to ensure good milk production. She also advocated using cooked bean sprouts wrapped in a towel to treat breast engorgement.

While the literature reports that seaweed soup and rice are the only foods believed not to be harmful for the postpartum woman,[2,3] Younghee disagrees with this premise. In fact she advocates including acorn squash in the daily diet to relieve post-partum edema. To her, as long as the food is warm and soft, it can be eaten.

Younghee discussed the Korean proscription against bathing, washing hair, and brushing teeth during the postpartum period, but considers these taboos to be "nasty" and does not adhere to them. "As long as the water is warm and the new mother does not get cold, it is okay to bathe. She needs to be clean." She is supportive of helping a postpartum woman to rest and spend time with her baby.

Younghee was able to recall the births of her younger siblings in Korea. She stated that her mother had delivered her children at home. "A midwife would come and us kids would be put in the kitchen or living area. We were not allowed in the bedroom while mother was giving birth. But, even though this was not the usual custom, my father would go in and help the midwife when the time for the birth came, because there was no one else to help her. It would grow very quiet in the bedroom and then we would hear the baby crying. Most babies are born in hospitals in Korea now, and fathers are not allowed to attend the birth."

This interview demonstrates how culture and personal experience can influence an individual's beliefs and practices. It is, thus, important for health care workers to make cultural assessment a part of their total client evaluation and to individualize their interventions.

Recipe for Seaweed Soup

Ingredients
2 feet of dry seaweed
1/2 pound sea mussels (rinsed)
Clove of garlic or garlic powder to taste
Salt to taste or soy sauce to taste
Water

Directions
Soak seaweed in warm water for 1 hour. In a pot, sauté sea mussels in a small amount of vegetable oil (just enough to prevent sticking). Add soaked seaweed, garlic, and salt or soy sauce. Add enough water to cover all ingredients and bring to boil. Simmer for 20 minutes. This makes enough soup for approximately 10 bowls of seaweed soup. The dried seaweed is obtainable in some supermarkets and in Korean grocery stores.

References

1. Microsoft Encarta 96 Encyclopedia (1993–1995). Korea. Funk and Wagnalls Corporation

2. Howard JY, Berbiglia VA. Caring for childbearing Korean women. *J Obstet Gynecol Neonatal Nurs.* 1997;26:665–671

3. Han YJ, Do SR, Park JH, Lee SO. *Study on Mortality Rate and Cause of Death.* Seoul, Korea: Korea Institute for Health and Social Affairs; 1996

4. Office of Statistics (Korea). *Korean Annual Statistical Report, No. 41.* Seoul, Korea: National Statistical Office, Korean Institute for Health and Social Affairs; 1994

5. Choi EC. The unique aspects of Korean-American mothers. *J Obstet Gynecol Neonatal Nurs.* 1986;15:394–400

6. Johnson RC, Bowman KS, Schwitters SY, Nagoshi CT, Wilson JR, Parks JY. Ethnic, familial, and environmental influences on lactose intolerance. *Human Biology.* 1984;56:307–316

7. Lim JK, Hwang NM, Chang DH. *Study on Maternal and Child Health Program Evaluation in the Urban Area.* Seoul, Korea: Korean Institute for Health and Social Affairs; 1991

8. Yang JM. Study on the Korean family planning situation and problems. *J Prev Med.* 1991;24:70–85

Further Reading

Choi YH. Issues on women's health. In: *Report from the Women's Health Promotion Center Opening Symposium: Women's Health and Human Rights.* Seoul, Korea: College of Nursing, Ewha Woman's University; 1998

Choi YS, Ko MS, Lee KE, Kim SY. Study on women's health for violence, sexual abuse, divorce cases. *J Korean Women Health Nurs Acad Soc.* 1996;2:92–107

Han IR. Study on the incidence of the unmarried mother and trend of the welfare of the unmarried mother. *3rd Korean Matern Child Health Mem Acad Rep.* 1998

Kim ES. Role of women: view of anthropology. *1st Korean Matern Child Health.* Establishment Memorial Acad Workshop Rep 1996:77–83

Lee KH. Conceptual model for women's health. *J Korean Acad Nurs.* 1997;27:933–942

Lee KH. Identity of women's health nursing. *1st Korean Women Health Nurs Acad Soc.* 1998;4:29–37

Lee KH. Issue of women's health. *Korean J Nurs Query.* 1996;5:39–58

Pang S. Trend on the maternal and child health situation. *1st Korean Matern Child Health Mem Acad Rep.* 1996:17–76

Park JH. Promotion of maternal and child health and family planning. In: *26th Health Day Memorial Symposium Report.* Seoul, Korea: Korean Public Health Association; 1998

Report from the Women's Health Promotion Center Opening Memorial Symposium: Women's Health and Human Rights. Seoul, Korea: College of Nursing, Ewha Woman's University; 1998

Yang JM. Study on the Korean family planning situation and problems. *J Prev Med.* 1991;24:70–85

11
Perinatal Health Care Issues of Mexican Women

Leonora Calsada and Patricia Lozada-Santone

Mexicans are not a homogeneous group of people. The population can be classified as indigenous European, Asian, African, or some combination thereof.[1] Mexican immigrants represent the largest group of working poor in the United States.[2] Very few are college educated, more than half do not obtain their high school diploma, most do not speak English, and a significant number are functionally illiterate in English and Spanish.[3] Recent data indicate that 26.6% of Hispanics in the United States live below the poverty level.[2]

Mexicans who have entered the United States illegally experience significant hardship and trauma. They make many sacrifices to enter this country and usually are not prepared for the realities they encounter, including discrimination and prejudice, substandard living conditions, and communities that are often crime-ridden and drug-infested. The occupations that many Mexicans hold are low paying and involve significant physical labor. These menial jobs seldom provide health insurance or any other benefits.

Health and Illness

Many issues affect the reproductive health care needs of Mexican women. Language, culture, lack of monetary resources, undocumented residency status, and inadequate medical coverage often prevent access to health care services in the United States.[4,5] Even when medical care is accessible, a clash often exists between the beliefs traditionally held by Mexicans and those espoused by the Western health care system.[6]

Culturally and spiritually, a significant number of Mexicans may have difficulty accepting the biomedical model of health care practiced in the United States. Instead, many Mexican families prefer to consult an older and wiser family member (usually a woman) for advice, remedies, or cures when someone in the family is ill. When an illness is beyond this particular individual's knowledge, an outsider's help may be sought.[7]

There are many components that play a part in the Mexican folk health care system, including the beliefs associated with the ideas about the nature of the world. There is a strong and pervasive belief in the balance of nature and the fatalistic belief that "God's will" always prevails. There are also many taboos associated with the qualities of "hot" and "cold" as is true of many Asian cultures. Heat and coldness can affect health, illness, and conditions such as pregnancy. When the balance is disrupted, a person becomes ill. The most common practice used to restore balance and/or to cure an ill person involves the use of herbal cures, sometimes described as the practice of "green medicine." Herbal cures are part of the elaborate system of folk healing that Mexicans and Mexican Americans refer to as *curanderismo*.[8,9]

Curanderismo refers to the act of curing and is derived from the Spanish verb *curar* (to cure). A practitioner or a healer is known as a *curandero*. There are various types of *curanderos*: *espiritistas* are individuals who enter a medium between this world and the spirits, *parteras* are women who care for pregnant women and deliver babies, *señoras* are women who foretell the future by reading cards, *yerberos* are individuals who are well-versed in the use of herbal cures, and *sobadores/sobadoras* are individuals who practice the art of massage.[10,11]

The health care provider must understand and acknowledge the traditional health practices of Mexicans to be more culturally sensitive and less likely to label them as noncompliant. Generally speaking, when providing medical care for the Mexican patient, the provider should be cognizant of 3 factors. First, Mexicans will readily render respect, even to non-authority figures; however, there is an expectation of reciprocity. A patient will likely not return for medical care if respect is lacking or not sincerely expressed. Second, a Mexican patient does not usually make decisions without consulting with the family. Indeed, family opinion is often more valuable than individual opinion. Thus a provider should attempt to include family members in prevention and treatment plans. Furthermore, Mexicans tend to stress the importance of *personalismo,* or personal rather than impersonal relationships. A Mexican patient will tend to develop a relationship with the provider instead of the organization or institution. Thus it is important for the provider to express interest in the patient as a person,[12] and, when possible, continuity of care and follow-up should be provided by the same caregiver.

Pregnancy/Prenatal Care

Mexicans tend to view pregnancy as a pleasant and positive experience. Moreover, many women state they feel healthiest when they are pregnant. The Mexican community is very protective of the pregnant woman because she is perceived as vulnerable. As such, she usually receives more attention from her spouse, family, and friends while pregnant than before or after pregnancy. Her own mother tends to become more involved in her pregnancy as the time for birth approaches.

The delivery of prenatal care to Mexican women requires a thorough understanding of their cultural and religious backgrounds. Female providers are generally preferred. Mexican women are often too polite to disagree with health care providers and may verbally agree to recommendations that they will never follow. However, they tend to be more compliant with advice that is provided by those who are bilingual/bicultural, and may be more forthcoming in revealing personal information to them.

In Mexico, pregnancy is not considered to be a state of illness; rather, it is viewed as a natural part of the life cycle. Many Mexican women do not seek prenatal care early in their pregnancy simply because they feel healthy. Thus prenatal care is usually initiated solely to confirm a pregnancy and to determine an estimated date of delivery. Their mothers and the older women in their families and community generally provide advice and guidance throughout their pregnancy and during the postpartum period.[13] Many pregnant women will only seek medical attention if a problem develops; otherwise, they will simply return when they are in labor.

Initiating prenatal care in the United States may be further complicated for Mexican women by inadequate or lack of medical insurance; insufficient financial resources to pay for health services; logistical factors, such as transportation; other traditional demands that are considered more important (eg, maintaining household, caring for children, etc); language; inconvenient hours of service; long waits in providers' offices, long waits to get an appointment; lack of child care services; cost of prenatal care; loss of pay from work when absent for appointments; and fear of connections between providers and immigration authorities. All of these barriers can influence actual compliance with medical care.[14]

Although Mexican women often want to know the gender of the baby, they really do not have a gender preference. What is considered most important is the health of the baby. Women will meet with genetic counselors when advised to do so by their health care providers; however, they are quite hesitant to consent to procedures such as amniocentesis because they often fear having a miscarriage following the procedure. However, ultrasonography is not considered invasive and is, thus, acceptable. In fact, once prenatal care is established, the Mexican patient often expects to have an ultrasound, and if she does not have one, she may believe she is receiving substandard medical care.

Blood tests can be anxiety provoking to Mexican women. They almost always question why the specimen needs to be taken and how much blood must be drawn; they perceive the test to be invasive and are uneasy with having any amount taken. Mexican women do not readily accept the notion that one's body can replenish the blood that is removed or lost and believe that they will be weakened by any loss. This anxiety and fear of blood tests can also stem from the common practice of threatening children with injections when they misbehave.

Elective abortion tends to be unacceptable to Mexicans, even when a problem or an anomaly is identified. There is a strong belief that the status of the fetus can change if God so desires or *"si Dios quiere."* Thus to consent to an abortion implies disbelief in God's ultimate power. Often believing it is a sin, a Mexican woman who does undergo an abortion may experience a significant degree of unresolved feelings, including guilt, self-blame, and depression. If for whatever reason a Mexican woman decides to terminate her pregnancy, she may use a strong herbal tea to induce abortion; likewise, she may use herbal teas to prevent a miscarriage.

It is not uncommon for a Mexican woman to never have undergone a gynecologic examination before pregnancy. Pelvic examinations are often viewed as invasive and may, thus, be a deterrent toward initiating prenatal care. The Mexican male partner is also very uneasy with this examination, especially if done by a male provider. The health care provider must be sensitive to this and discuss its importance before proceeding with the history and physical examination.

Mexican women often do not perceive themselves as being at risk for sexually transmitted diseases (STDs) and human immunodeficiency virus (HIV) because they are generally monogamous and faithful to their partners. Even when they do consent to STD and HIV testing, they do not expect to have positive results. They generally have difficulty accepting possible infidelity by their partners, and they will not readily admit it, even when they are aware of it.

Pregnant Mexican women are encouraged to eat regularly; avoid alcohol consumption and tobacco exposure, including smoking and secondhand smoke; and avoid the use of any kind of addictive substance or drug. Eating fruits, vegetables, and soups is encouraged. They are often urged to eat whatever they crave, and are discouraged from eating irregularly or missing meals. Some Mexican women crave soil substances such as dirt, mud, or clay, a very dangerous practice because of possible lead and chemical exposures. Women often avoid eating big, greasy meals and believe they will experience stomach upset or *empacho* if this is done. Generally, women are not concerned with excessive weight gain and often believe that their baby will be healthier if they are not thin or underweight. Body image concerns or issues are not commonly observed, although more attention is placed on body cleanliness and having neat or clean clothing during pregnancy.

There is a strong belief in the need to avoid having any strong emotional reactions while pregnant. An intense reaction is believed to have adverse effects on the fetus. Women are urged by family members and concerned friends to especially avoid situations that provoke fear, or *susto*, which is commonly believed to cause preterm labor and delivery or miscarriage. Mexican women are also advised to not experience intense anger, or *hacer coraje*. This too is believed to affect a pregnancy outcome.

Beliefs about sexual intimacy vary; however, there is a general belief that it is best to avoid intercourse late in pregnancy. Often, Mexican men avoid sex with their wives because they are convinced it will harm the baby. Pregnant women avoid crossing their legs while sitting because they believe this will cause fetal strangulation.

It is believed that a fetus exposed to a lunar eclipse will be born with malformations such as a cleft lip or a deformed extremity. Women protect the unborn by using safety pins on clothing and/or by fastening a piece of red cloth to their intimate apparel.

Labor and Delivery

Many Mexican women living in the United States accept their partner's presence during birth. Some, however, still express being uncomfortable and embarrassed, preferring to have their mothers or other female relatives present instead. Mexican women are very modest and appreciate having their privacy respected.

Although some women will enroll in birthing classes, most do not believe it is necessary because labor and delivery are viewed as natural events requiring little if any preparation. Mexican women tend to feel very confident with the birthing process and do not expect to experience any complications; men generally believe classes review information that is considered a "woman's business." Very few couples attend classes.

Most Mexican women prefer natural childbirth and fear that pain medication, including epidurals, may have adverse effects on themselves as well as the baby. Many take pride in being able to withstand and tolerate the pain of childbirth and may receive recognition and praise from their significant others for their endurance. During labor, it is not uncommon for Mexican women to want to eat, and it is difficult for them to understand why they should not consume any food during this time. They are very uncomfortable with practices that they perceive as unnatural, such as routine intravenous hydration. However, they will generally accept a heparin lock to keep the vein open. Although choices for labor positioning vary from individual to individual, being confined to bed in a supine position is usually not desirable, as is having frequent vaginal examinations. In labor, a Mexican woman is not admonished from making noises and, thus, may be very expressive. A hospital delivery is generally preferred over a home birth because it is often perceived as a status symbol.

Postpartum and Newborn Care

The postpartum period is commonly called *la cuarentena.* For 40 days the Mexican woman is believed to be vulnerable and susceptible to many ailments. She is, thus, expected to maintain a sedentary disposition and is advised to *reposar,* or rest, as she recovers. The new mother is not expected to involve herself in any strenuous physical activity and is helped extensively by other female family members with maintaining her usual household responsibilities. It is believed that she will experience *caida de la matriz,* or prolapsed uterus, if she engages in significant physical activity. To enhance uterine involution, some women will use medicinal compresses on their abdomens during the early postpartum period. Other women will use a girdle, or *faja,* to protect the uterus. Sexual intercourse is commonly avoided during this period.

Tub baths during *la cuarentena* also are viewed as harmful. While showering is more preferable, some women will only practice "towel bathing" during this period. This is because of their adherence to the "hot" and "cold" belief. Personal hygiene is so important that some woman overuse vaginal lavage or douching treatments after giving birth. The postpartum diet is very important, especially if a woman is breastfeeding her infant. She often will eat soups, avoid spicy foods, and basically eat light meals. The consumption of high-caloric shakes, or *atoles,* which are hot shakes, is quite common during lactation, as is the occasional consumption of beer to increase the quality and quantity of breast milk. Infant colic is believed to be caused by the foods ingested by the mother. Mexican women are generally aware of the benefits of breastfeeding; however, it is not always the preferred method for infant feeding. Increasingly, some women perceive bottle-feeding as a more modern method, representing an enhancement in social status.

Care of the newborn is almost exclusively the woman's responsibility, with men participating minimally; however, this is changing gradually because of the exposure to American mainstream practices. Due to their "hot" and "cold" beliefs, some Mexican women are hesitant to bathe their infant during the first few weeks of life, believing that it will cause a disharmony.

The infant's umbilicus is cared for fastidiously. It is usually cleaned with cotton balls and baby or cooking oils. An infant is not allowed to cry for any long period because this is believed to cause a hernia in the umbilicus. Many women use what is called a *fajero,* or girdlelike strap, around the infant's belly to protect the umbilicus. A protruding umbilicus is considered abnormal, and when this does occur, it is believed to result from poor care. Much attention is also placed on the care of the infant's fontanel. Anyone holding the baby will avoid sudden movements or shaking, as this is believed to cause *caida de mollera,* or fallen fontanel. It is also believed that this will occur when a nipple is pulled or removed suddenly from an infant's mouth.

Many infant ailments such as skin rashes, diarrhea, constipation, and vomiting are initially treated with home remedies. If they are not successful, mothers then seek medical care. However, mothers seldom seek medical care for folk illnesses such as *empacho* or *caida de mollera.*

Infant colic is acknowledged as occurring frequently, and numerous strategies are practiced to avoid it. For example, a breastfeeding woman will usually make changes in her diet and will avoid *susto* or *coraje* because they are believed to spoil her milk and make the baby colicky. Additionally, herbal teas are commonly used by mothers and often given to infants as well. Attention must be paid to this practice because sometimes the teas may be used to substitute entire infant feedings.

Generally speaking, circumcision is not acceptable; however, if the father has been circumcised, the baby will probably have the procedure performed as well. As for baby girls, it is a very common practice to have their ears pierced soon after birth.

Great care is taken to protect the baby from the natural elements. It is not uncommon for new mothers to overdress their babies because of their belief in *mal aire,* or bad air. This practice is associated with a concern about airborne contaminants, and new mothers may need to be instructed about its inherent dangers. Besides the concern with the natural elements, there is also a significant concern with unintentional harm being caused by individuals. It is believed that an individual can cause harm to an infant through staring with admiration and awe. This phenomenon is known as *mal de ojo,* or evil eye. Preventive measures include adorning infants with bracelets and necklaces. Another preventive measure is for the admirer to touch the head of the infant being complimented or admired.

There are no common rituals that are attached to the naming of a child. However, if the family is very traditional, the child's last name will include the mother's and father's surnames. It is not uncommon to choose the name of a saint, especially if the child is born on a day dedicated to a particular saint. Baptism is the one sacrament that is almost universally practiced. It is widely believed that babies must be baptized soon after birth to protect their spirits should illness or death occur.

Family Planning

Mexican women tend to view birth control injectibles as a convenient, nonintrusive, and uncomplicated method of contraception. Oral contraceptives are less acceptable because of the potential side effects of weight gain, mood changes, increased facial pigmentation, and possible infertility. Depending on their religious beliefs, some will accept the use of an intrauterine device (IUD). The diaphragm is generally disliked because it requires self-touching of the genitals. Some women rely on breastfeeding for family planning. Female sterilization is an acceptable method of birth control if and when the woman and her partner have had as many children as they desire. However, some women fear bilateral tubal ligation because of the possibility of complications following the procedure. The psychological implications of sterilization for a traditional Mexican woman can be devastating because she may view the ability to procreate as a significant aspect of her identity as a woman.

Birth control is traditionally considered a woman's responsibility. Because the use of condoms requires the man's participation, this form of birth control is not frequently used. Some Mexican men continue to manifest traits associated with machismo, or male chauvinistic behavior.

Death/Burial Rites

Mexican women generally have uncomplicated adjustments to pregnancy losses because of their strong belief that it is a result of God's intervention and not the fault of the woman. When a fetal death occurs, some women like to view, hold, and take pictures, and save a lock of the baby's hair. It is not uncommon for the baby to be named, and for the woman to believe that the baby ascended to heaven. Families prefer to bury the infant; however, sometimes because of monetary constraints, cremation is chosen.

Every Mexican Woman Is Unique

Practices, beliefs, and behaviors will vary from individual to individual, and providers should not expect all Mexicans to ascribe to a stereotypical pattern.[15] Thus attempts to assess the actual degree of acculturation and assimilation with the American way of life will help to make the delivery of medical care more relevant and appropriate for the individual Mexican woman. Mexican women must be seen on a continuum in relation to their degree of acculturation in the United States. Perinatal health care providers need to be aware that at one end of the continuum are those women who are traditional. They have the attributes of the historical Mexican culture, especially as rooted in rural, peasant origins, and that at the other end of the continuum are those women almost fully assimilated into US culture, with little left of their Mexican origins except for their Hispanic surnames. In the middle is the group often described as bicultural, but representing a range of adherence to tradition extending from the literal to the symbolic. In this group are those women simultaneously attempting to identify with the mainstream US culture while retaining elements of the cultural practices that make them distinctly Mexican. It is this group of women that is most frequently encountered by health care providers.

Perinatal Health Care Issues of Mexican Women: Key Highlights

Psychosocial/Spiritual Characteristics

- Mexicans tend to be respectful toward health care providers and expect reciprocity.
- They tend to believe, almost fatalistically, that God's will always prevails.
- Illness is often attributed to an imbalance of "hot" and "cold."
- Baptism is believed to protect the spirit of the baby in the event of illness or death.
- Older family members (usually females) are generally consulted for advice and/or remedies.

Prenatal Care

- Female health care providers are preferred.
- Women are more receptive to health care providers who are bilingual/bicultural.
- Prenatal care is usually sought in the second trimester.
- Compliance with prenatal care is often complicated by socioeconomic factors.

Prenatal Testing

- Mexican women tend to expect ultrasound testing.
- Amniocentesis may be feared; however, they are often amenable to genetic counseling.
- Routine blood testing causes apprehension.
- Abortion is often unacceptable, even when a problem or an anomaly is identified.
- Most hold a fatalistic belief that an anomaly is God's will.
- Traditional/religious women believe it is a mortal sin to have an abortion.
- Many are resistant to pelvic examination.

- Most women do not perceive themselves as being at risk for HIV and STDs. Testing is highly recommended because of the possibility that their partners may have had multiple sex partners.

Pregnancy Diet
- Mexican women tend to have a very healthy diet; however, excessive intake may be a problem.
- Alcohol, tobacco, and other drugs are usually avoided.
- Cravings for unusual and dangerous substances (eg, dirt, mud, clay, etc) may be observed.
- Eating big greasy meals is believed to cause a folk illness known as *empacho.*

Pregnancy-Related Beliefs/Taboos
- *Susto,* or fright, and *hacer coraje,* or intense anger, are folk conditions that are perceived to be harmful to the pregnancy.
- Sexual intimacy is generally avoided in late pregnancy; some men will avoid sex completely because they fear harming the baby.
- Some women avoid crossing their legs because of a belief that they will strangle the baby.
- Lunar eclipses are believed to be very harmful to the fetus.

Labor and Delivery
- Women prefer natural childbirth.
- Invasive routines such as intravenous hydration and frequent pelvic examinations are to be avoided, if possible.
- Women are permitted to be very expressive during labor.
- Labor positioning varies from individual to individual; however, many dislike the supine position.
- The hospital is the preferred site for birth; it is perceived as a status symbol.

Postpartum Care

- A 40-day recovery period, known as *la cuarentena,* is widely observed.
- Strenuous physical activity is avoided to prevent *caida de la matriz,* or prolapsed uterus.
- Abdominal medicinal compresses are frequently used to enhance uterine involution.
- Sexual intercourse is avoided during *la cuarentena.*
- Some women will wear girdles to protect the uterus.
- Taking a bath is viewed as harmful; showering or towel bathing is preferred.
- Douching is a common practice, and excessive use may be a problem.

Postpartum Diet

- Soups and light meals are preferred; spicy foods are avoided.

Neonatal Care

- Infant bathing is avoided during the first 2 weeks of life.
- Care of the infant's umbilicus is very important. An infant girdle-like strap called a *fajero* may be used.
- Care of the infant's fontanel is quite important; *caida de mollera,* or fallen fontanel, is of great concern.
- Care of colic may involve the use of medicinal teas.
- Home remedies are used to treat common infant illnesses (eg, skin rash, diarrhea, and constipation).
- Babies are protected from the natural elements by bundling them up.
- It is believed that individuals can cause unintentional harm through staring with admiration and awe.
- Circumcision is not usually accepted unless the father is circumcised.
- No common rituals are attached to the naming of a child.

- Traditional families will include both the father's and mother's surnames in the child's last name.
- A child will be named after a saint if born on a day dedicated to a particular saint.

Breastfeeding/Breast Care
- Diet is very important, especially if a woman is breastfeeding.
- Consumption of high-caloric shakes is recommended for breast-feeding.
- Occasionally beer will be consumed to increase the quantity and quality of breast milk.
- The benefits of breastfeeding are understood; however, it is not generally the preferred method.

Family Planning
- Birth control is considered a woman's responsibility.
- Women prefer birth control injections.
- Oral contraceptives are not generally acceptable.
- IUDs may be acceptable, depending on the woman's religious beliefs.
- The diaphragm is generally disliked.
- Breastfeeding is perceived as a birth control method by some women.
- Female sterilization may be acceptable.
- Condoms are not frequently used.

Family Involvement
- Female family members provide extensive emotional support, practical assistance, and guidance.
- The pregnant woman's mother is very involved, especially at the end of the pregnancy.
- Men are more involved during childbearing in the United States than in Mexico.
- Couples usually do not attend childbirth education classes.

- Newborn care is almost exclusively the woman's responsibility.
- Female family members assist the new mother when needed.

Pregnancy Termination/Miscarriage
- Mexicans tend to have a fatalistic belief that any loss is God's will.
- Viewing and holding a deceased infant is often desired.

Death/Burial Rites
- Burial is preferred; however, cremation may be chosen due to monetary constraints.

References

1. Goodrich JK. *The Coming of Mexico.* Chicago, IL: Plumpton Press; 1913
2. Hajat A, Lucas JB, Kington R. *Health Outcomes Among Hispanic Subgroups: Data From the National Health Interview Survey, 1992–1995.* Hyattsville, MD: National Center for Health Statistics; 2000. #310
3. US Department of Commerce, Bureau of Census. *October Current Population Survey.* Washington, DC: US Department of Commerce, Bureau of Census; 1996
4. Amaro H. Women in the Mexican-American community: religion, culture and reproductive attitudes and experiences. *J Community Psychol.* 1988;16:6–19
5. Joyce K, Diffenbacker G, Greene J, Sorakin Y. Internal and external barriers to obtaining prenatal care. *Soc Work Health Care.* 1993;9:89–96
6. Peña CC. *Provider Opinion of Causes of Low Neonatal Mortality Rate in Mexican and Mexican-American Populations in the United States* [master's thesis]. San Diego, CA: San Diego State University
7. Kiev A. *Curanderismo: Mexican-American Folk Psychiatry.* New York, NY: Free Press; 1972
8. Torres E. *Green Medicine: Traditional Mexican-American Herbal Remedies.* Kingsville, TX: Nieves Press; 1983
9. Rose LC. *Disease Beliefs in Mexican-American Communities.* San Francisco, CA: R & E Research Associates, Inc; 1978
10. Torres E. *The Folk Healer: The Mexican-American Tradition of Curanderismo.* Kingsville, TX: Nieves Press; 1983
11. Ford KC. *Las Yerbas de la Gente: A Study of Hispano-American Medicinal Plants.* Ann Arbor, MI: University of Michigan; 1975

12. COSSMHO. *The National Hispanic Prenatal Hotline: Maternal and Child Health MEMO.* Washington, DC: National Coalition of Hispanic Health and Human Services Organizations; 1998

13. Crispín AL, Rappsilber C. *Beliefs of the Pregnant Women Associated With Prenatal Care.* Washington, DC: National Institutes of Health; 1995. NIH Publication No. 98-4295

14. Jasis M. *Creencias y Tradiciones Sobre Salud Prenatal.* Tijuana, Baja, CA: Centro de Estudios Fronterizos de Norte de Mexico; 1985

15. Bock WR. *The Influence of Acculturation on Mexican Folk Health Beliefs and Practices* [master's thesis]. San Diego, CA: San Diego State University; 1987

12
Perinatal Health Care Issues
of Mormon Women

Lisa Jones Conley

Members of the Church of Jesus Christ of Latter-Day Saints (LDS) are called Mormons because their religion is based on a book of scripture called the Book of Mormon. Approximately 11 million people worldwide adhere to the LDS faith, with a large concentration in the state of Utah.[1] Marriage rates are higher among this group than among the general US population, and faithful Mormons who marry in their temples divorce only one fifth as often as the national average. Birth control and abortion rates are low in this culture, which accounts for the highest birth rate in the nation.[2] Today members of the Mormon faith maintain a fairly low profile within society. However, as contraception, abortion, divorce, and the sexual revolution become more mainstream in society, Mormonism has become viewed as an increasingly unusual culture.

During the early 19th century, the Eastern United States was troubled with religious unrest, and numerous sects of religion challenged one another in an effort to gain acceptance and stability. A young man named Joseph Smith, whose family lived in upstate New York, found himself caught up in the religious fervor. After much thought and deliberation, Joseph decided to ask God to find out for himself which of the many sects he should join, and in so doing, he received what Mormons call The First Vision. In this vision, God the Father and his Son, Jesus Christ, appeared to Joseph and answered his prayer. Joseph was instructed to join none of the existing religious sects. The Lord then explained that, due to corruption in the early Christian church,

Christ's true church had been taken from the earth. Joseph was to be the Lord's instrument in restoring His true church and gospel back to the earth.[3]

Religious History

A few years after his vision experience, Joseph was visited by an angel who revealed to him the location of a book made of gold plates on which were written the gospel of Jesus Christ and the history and religion of an ancient American people. These people were Israelites who had been led by the Lord to North America and whose descendants are the American Indians. The book includes information about the appearance and ministry of Jesus Christ to these people after His mortal ministry and resurrection in Jerusalem. With the guidance of the Lord, Joseph translated the writing on the plates into English; today this translation is known as the Book of Mormon and is accepted as an important second witness to the Bible of the divinity of Jesus Christ.

Joseph established the Church of Jesus Christ of Latter-Day Saints in 1830.[3] Many joined the newly established church, which incorporated into its religious code the ethical standards and basic doctrines of the New Testament, such as the golden rule; the necessity for good works, faith, repentance, and baptism; virtue; honor; and prayer. Mormons also believe in continuous modern-day revelation through a living prophet.

Almost from its inception, members of the Mormon Church were severely persecuted. Indeed, their founder and prophet, Joseph Smith, was murdered. To escape this persecution, the Mormons sought refuge in the western United States, and in 1847 Mormon pioneers established a home in the Great Salt Lake Valley of Utah. Here, they believed they could practice their religion without fear of persecution; however, persecution persisted as a result of their belief and practice of the doctrine of plural marriage.[3]

Polygamy had been established in the early Mormon Church as a commandment from the Lord. Contrary to popular thought, most Mormons resisted the practice of polygamy, and those who did practice it had to be called by church leaders and meet specific criteria. In 1890, the US Supreme Court ruled polygamy unconstitutional, and, subsequently, the church issued a manifesto that terminated its practice. Mormons continue to be linked with polygamy even though the doctrine was abolished and has not been practiced by them for more than 100 years.

To fully understand Mormon attitudes toward marriage, home, and family, one must first become familiar with some specific beliefs and practices. Mormons believe in the Godhead, which consists of 3 separate immortal beings: God the Father, His son Jesus Christ (both have physical, resurrected bodies of flesh and bone), and the Holy Ghost (a spiritual personage). All are believed to be in the form of man, and each speaks and has spoken to man. Each is all wise, all powerful, merciful, and kind.[4]

Mormons believe that all people are the spirit children of God the Father and Heavenly Mother and that all dwelt with them prior to this mortal existence. They believe that all of God's spirit children come into mortality, obtain a body, and learn to choose right from wrong through their own experiences. This they call the Plan of Salvation, through which all may return to God through the atonement of Jesus Christ and obedience to His commandments.[4] Mormon doctrine sets forth standards to which faithful members conform and adhere. They live by these standards every minute of every day and dedicate their lives to building the Kingdom of God on the earth.[4]

Mormons define the priesthood as the power and authority to act in the name of God. The priesthood allows Mormon men to preside in the Church and in the home. Every worthy Mormon male from the age of 12 years can receive the priesthood, which is conferred in successive stages, each providing a higher degree of responsibility.

Priesthood authority is required to perform such ordinances as temple marriage, birth blessings (christening), the ordinance of the sacrament, healings, and baptism. The Mormon father, if worthy, performs most of the religious ordinances for his family that a minister or priest might perform for members of other Christian denominations. Mormons claim direct priesthood authority from God. They believe the priesthood was lost after the death of Christ's apostles because of corruption in the early Christian church, and that the priesthood was restored to Joseph Smith and others through ministering angels sent from the Lord.[4]

The Word of Wisdom is a doctrine encompassing the belief that the body is the home of the spirit and should be kept holy and pure. The Word of Wisdom states that members should not consume coffee, tea, tobacco, alcohol, illegal drugs, or any other harmful or addictive substance, and purity should be sought physically, mentally, and spiritually.[5] Mormonism is a religious culture that significantly affects every aspect of its members' lives.

The Mormon Temple is a holy building where religious ordinances are performed. Because of the sacred nature of the building, only faithful Mormon members are permitted to enter. According to their theology, a couple or family can be "sealed" together forever in the temple by the power and authority of the priesthood. They believe that temple sealings allow for family relationships to be perpetuated beyond the grave.[6] Each faithful Mormon who has participated in sacred ordinances in the temple receives an article of clothing called a "temple garment." It is worn daily by faithful members throughout their lives and is considered sacred and holy.

Marriage is highly valued in Mormonism and is believed to be essential to God's eternal plan.[6] Mormons believe that God instituted marriage for the establishment and preservation of family life and so that the spiritual and physical needs of children can be met. For these reasons, divorce is strongly discouraged, and Mormons are counseled to work diligently in keeping their families intact.[4] Marriage in God's temple creates an eternal family unit and is believed to be one of the greatest blessings Mormons can obtain in this life. Children born to a couple married in the temple are said to be "born in the covenant" and are sealed to their parents forever. Thus a popular slogan in the church is "families are forever."

Mormon members accept certain roles and responsibilities specific to their gender. They believe that "gender is an essential characteristic of individual premortal, mortal, and eternal identity and purpose."[6] The Mormon family structure is patriarchal. The father presides over the family in love and righteousness. He is the spiritual and actual head of the home and is responsible for providing the necessities of life and protection for his family. Mothers are primarily responsible for bearing children and nurturing them. In carrying out these sacred responsibilities, fathers and mothers are obligated to help one another as equal partners.[6]

In Mormonism, motherhood is honored, respected, and revered as a godly calling. Motherhood is considered equal to the male role of priesthood bearer and is considered to be the most important aspect of a woman's life. Mormon females are reared to be wives, mothers, and homemakers, and once they have children, they are urged to make motherhood a career. "She who rears successfully a family of healthy, beautiful sons and daughters, whose influence will be felt through generations to come…deserves the highest honors that man can give, and the choicest blessings of God."[7]

Mormons believe that "the sacred powers of procreation are to be used only between husband and wife."[6] Physical intimacy is a sacred expression of love within marriage. Sexual activities outside of marriage are in direct violation of God's laws, and anyone who participates in them is subject to church discipline. Virginity is held in high esteem for non-married men and women alike.

Mormons are dramatically more conservative than the rest of the nation regarding premarital sexual norms. A study conducted at Brigham Young University[8] found the youth that were taught and lived gospel principles, regardless of where they lived, held firmly to the ideal of chastity. Most disapproved of and did not engage in petting, masturbation, or homosexual behaviors, and intercourse was considered more serious than any other behavior.[8] Mormonism teaches strict premarital chastity. If a female becomes pregnant outside of wedlock, it is a distressing situation for the individuals involved as well as their families. The preferred choices in these circumstances are either marriage of the individuals involved or placement of the infant up for adoption. Therapeutic abortions are against church doctrine and, therefore, are not an option.[4,9] Post-marital fidelity is strictly observed; adultery is considered a grievous sin—nearly equivalent to murder—and is grounds for excommunication from the church.[9] Homosexuality is also regarded as sinful and counter to God's eternal plan.[4,6,9]

Adolescent or unwed mothers frequently experience guilt at becoming pregnant outside of marriage. Often they will place the infant up for adoption and almost always will request a Mormon family to receive the child. When adoption is indicated, LDS Family Services (which can be found under Church of Jesus Christ of Latter-Day Saints in the white pages) can be contacted for placement of the infant.

Health and Illness

Health care providers should strive to understand the implications that Mormon beliefs and practices have on perinatal care issues in order to provide holistic care to Mormon families. They should be mindful that information should be given with both husband and wife present because important family decisions are made jointly, and that Mormons often process information in spiritual terms and make decisions through prayer. Health care providers may not always understand or agree with these decisions; but they must always be respectful of them.

Any requests for priesthood blessing should be given priority. The priesthood holders should be given the opportunity to give such a blessing to the mother or infant, even when inconvenient. A priesthood blessing often provides more comfort to the family than medical interventions, and privacy during these blessings should always be respected. If a blessing is requested and there are no immediate priesthood holders available, a call can be made over the hospital intercom system requesting any LDS Elders to contact the hospital operator. Generally, this will produce results. When giving a healing blessing, the Elders (male priesthood holders) anoint the individual with a small amount of olive oil, which they usually bring with them. However, it is wise to keep a small container of olive oil on hand. Most premature or sick neonates will be given a birth blessing and commonly several healing blessings while in the neonatal intensive care unit.

Pregnancy/Prenatal Care

In Mormon childbearing practices, menstruation is felt to be a natural and necessary function that signifies the rights and blessings of womanhood. Only when a Mormon woman marries should she become pregnant, and solely as a result of sexual relations with her husband. Once married, she may become pregnant as often as desired throughout her reproductive years, a parity of 8 or more is not uncommon.

During pregnancy, it is the mother's responsibility to nourish and care for the developing body of the unborn spirit. This is accomplished through strict adherence to the Word of Wisdom and prenatal care. The physician/obstetrician is the principal caregiver during pregnancy, although midwives are becoming increasingly popular. An ultrasound of the fetus is generally desirable to evaluate the well-being and development of the fetus. However, prenatal testing for chromosomal or other abnormalities is not usually necessary. A therapeutic abortion in the event of an abnormality would not be likely.

Mormon women maintain great faith in the priesthood and often call on their husbands or other worthy priesthood holders to give them blessings for health, strength, and perseverance throughout their pregnancies. Such blessings are beneficial to the psychological and physical well-being of the mother.[10]

Infertility is a very distressing situation for members of this family-centered religion, and most infertile Mormon couples will seek medical assistance to attain pregnancy. Acceptable medical procedures for infertility are those that use the couple's own sperm and eggs. Sperm or egg donations, cloning, and surrogate motherhood all are strongly discouraged.[9]

Labor and Delivery

Labor is looked on as a natural process that should occur at the end of the ninth month. Most Mormon women adhere to the prevalent medical model of physician and hospital care for delivery, and most couples will allow as many medical procedures as necessary to produce a healthy infant. The delivery position is presumably the one most desired by the physician. During the labor process, the Mormon woman may wish to remain in her temple garments right up until the delivery of the infant. The husband is usually with his wife during the labor and delivery process; siblings and extended family members may also be in attendance.

Postpartum and Newborn Care

The postpartum period is one of recuperation and recovery for the Mormon mother. Extended family and church members are often very much involved in this period. They provide sibling care, meals, housework, and other daily necessities until the mother can manage on her own.

Circumcision is not a religious requirement in Mormon theology. Most Mormon male infants are circumcised because it is an accepted medical procedure rather than a religious requirement.[11]

An important ordinance takes place shortly after the birth of a child into a Mormon family. This ordinance consists of a priesthood blessing during which the child is named and given a blessing. The ordinance is most often pronounced by the infant's father, but must be given by a worthy priesthood holder. A premature or sick neonate would most likely have a birth blessing shortly after delivery, especially if his or her life is at risk. The birth blessing can provide great comfort to the family. It allows them to name and bless the infant, recognize the infant as an official member of their family, and acknowledge God and His blessings.

Most Mormon women believe that breast milk is superior to formula and view breastfeeding as important for the physical and emotional growth and development of the infant. The loss of the ability to breastfeed is often distressing to a Mormon mother. If an infant is born sick or premature, most Mormon mothers are diligent in pumping and saving their breast milk and will be adamant in its use whenever possible. The initiation of breastfeeding as soon as possible is highly recommended for a Mormon mother because it can provide her more control over her infant's care and facilitate bonding.

Family Planning

Mormon views on birth control and therapeutic abortions stem from their belief that all of God's children must come into mortality. With many spirits waiting for the opportunity to have an earthly body, it is paramount that Mormon couples provide for as many of these spirits as they are emotionally and physically able. Mormons believe that God's commandment to Adam and Eve to "multiply and replenish the earth" (Genesis 1:28) remains in effect.[6] Mormon couples are given their agency to determine their own family planning—believing that God will guide them in their choices.

Therapeutic abortions are forbidden in Mormonism, and those who obtain an abortion are subject to church discipline. In the event of rape, incest, and morbidity with a high probability of maternal death, a therapeutic abortion may be considered, but only on deep reflection and prayer and with the guidance of church leaders.[4,9]

Death/Burial Rites

When a fetus is lost through a spontaneous abortion or stillbirth, the Mormon family is greatly grieved for the loss of that spirit into their earthly family. They often find comfort from their belief that the lost child will be part of their eternal family.[4] If the family desires, they should be allowed to see and hold the deceased fetus, and they may wish to take the body home to be buried close to loved ones. With the loss of a pregnancy, the family, particularly the mother, feels a great loss. Commonly, another pregnancy quickly ensues.

In Mormonism, the life of a sick or premature infant often takes on religious significance. The infant is perceived as a choice and special spirit, and his or her life is held in high esteem. If he is "allowed" to live, the child is often felt to be preserved to fulfill some important earthly mission. If the infant dies, it is generally felt that he was an exceptionally righteous spirit who did not need the experiences of mortality and that his spirit has returned to God.

Mormon families who experience the death of an infant often find solace in 2 gospel principles. First, Mormons believe that children who die before the age of 8 years (age of accountability) immediately return to God. Second, Mormons believe that through a marriage that has been temple blessed, they have been sealed as an eternal family unit and, if they remain worthy, will be reunited with the child in the hereafter.[5]

Perinatal Health Care Issues of Mormon Women:
Key Highlights

Psychosocial/Spiritual Characteristics

- The family is the fundamental unit of the church.
- Religious practices play a significant part in everyday life.
- Strict premarital chastity and marital fidelity are stressed.
- Marriage between man and woman is ordained by God and essential to His eternal plan.
- Procreation is a sacred duty.

Prenatal Care

- Procedures for infertility are acceptable when using a husband's sperm and a wife's ova.
- Sperm and egg donation, cloning, and surrogate motherhood are strongly discouraged.
- Prenatal care is desirable.

Prenatal Testing

- Ultrasonography is acceptable to determine fetal well-being.
- Prenatal testing for chromosomal or other abnormalities is usually unnecessary because abortion is unlikely.

Labor and Delivery

- Most Mormon women adhere to the prevalent medical model of physician and hospital care for delivery.
- Most couples will allow as many medical procedures as necessary to produce a healthy infant.
- Analgesia and anesthesia are acceptable.
- The husband is usually with his wife during the labor and delivery process.
- Siblings and extended family members may also be in attendance.

Postpartum Care
- A period of recuperation and recovery is encouraged for the mother.

Neonatal Care
- Circumcision is not a religious requirement; however, many male infants are circumcised because it is an accepted medical procedure.
- The father and siblings take part in newborn care.
- Naming and birth blessing generally occurs within the first month. If the infant is sick or premature, it should take place shortly after birth.

Breastfeeding/Breast Care
- Breastfeeding is important both physically and psychologically for mother and infant.
- Breast milk is felt to be superior to formula.

Family Planning
- Contraception is an individual decision for each family.

Family Involvement
- The father or other family members often come to prenatal visits, and usually are in attendance during labor and delivery.
- Extended family and church members provide sibling care, meals, housework, and other daily necessities until the mother can manage on her own.

Pregnancy Termination/Miscarriage
- Therapeutic abortions are forbidden except in cases of rape, incest, or morbidity with a high probability of maternal death.

Death/Burial Rites
- Miscarriage is a tragedy for the family, especially the mother; the grieving parents are allowed to see and hold the deceased fetus if desired.

- Family should be allowed to take the body home to be buried close to loved ones if desired.
- Burial is not a religious requirement.
- Most families will have a ceremony and burial on the death of a preterm or term infant who lives beyond birth.

References

1. Church of Jesus Christ of Latter-Day Saints. *Conference Report.* Salt Lake City, UT: Church of Jesus Christ of Latter-Day Saints; 1999
2. Live births by race and Hispanic origin of mother: United States, each State and Territory, Preliminary 2000, and birth and fertility rates, final 1999 and preliminary 2000;49(5). Table 4. Available at: http://www.cdec.gov/nchs. Accessed July 22, 2003
3. Smith J. *History of the Church of Jesus Christ of Latter-Day Saints.* 2nd ed. Salt Lake City, UT: Deseret Book Co; 1963
4. The Church of Jesus Christ of Latter-Day Saints. Available at: http://www.lds.org. Accessed July 22, 2003
5. Church of Jesus Christ of Latter-Day Saints. *The Doctrine and Covenants of the Church of Jesus Christ of Latter-Day Saints.* Church of Jesus Christ of Latter-Day Saints. Salt Lake City, UT: Church of Jesus Christ of Latter-Day Saints; 1988
6. Church of Jesus Christ of Latter-Day Saints. *The Declaration on the Family.* Salt Lake City, UT: Church of Jesus Christ of Latter-Day Saints; 1997
7. McKay DO. Gospel ideals. In: *Improvement Era.* Salt Lake City, UT: Church of Jesus Christ of Latter-Day Saints; 1958
8. Top BL, Chadwick BA. *Helping Teens Stay Strong.* Salt Lake City, UT: Church of Jesus Christ of Latter-Day Saints; 1999
9. Church of Jesus Christ of Latter-Day Saints. *Official Priesthood Handbook.* Salt Lake City, UT: Church of Jesus Christ of Latter-Day Saints; 1999
10. Conley LJ. Childbearing and child rearing practices in Mormonism. *Neonatal Network.* 1990;9:41–47
11. Church of Jesus Christ of Latter-Day Saints. *The Book of Mormon: Another Testament of Jesus Christ.* Salt Lake City, UT: Church of Jesus Christ of Latter-Day Saints; 1981

13
Perinatal Health Care Issues of Native American Women: Tribes of the Northern Plains and Great Basin

Judy Edwards

Within the borders of the United States, including Alaska, 2.4 million American Indians reside as members of approximately 500 federally recognized tribes. While progress has been made in some areas, the overall mortality of American Indians is still 30% greater than for all races. And for selected causes, Indian mortality rates significantly exceed rates for all other races; for example, the accident rate is 310% greater, diabetes mellitus is 330% greater, tuberculosis is 530% greater, and liver disease/cirrhosis is 440% greater when compared with all races within the United States. The most recent data for 1993 reveals an Indian infant mortality rate of 10.9 per 1,000 live births compared, with 8.4 for all races.[1]

Tribal leaders report close to 40% of all Alaskan native households and 25% of Navajo households lack potable water and sanitary sewer systems.[1] The threats of a once nomadic life have been replaced by being a forgotten people in light of federal health programs, minimal economic development opportunities, and overwhelming poverty.

Health and Illness

Although once the dominant culture of this continent, very little is understood by non-Indian health providers about the health practices of the American Indian/Alaskan Native. There is still a common belief that the US government provides all the care that is needed and others have no reason to be concerned. It is true that through the treaties signed with the US government, tribes have secured health benefits. Unfortunately, the level of need and the degree of coverage was not included in the treaty language and Congress has never seen fit to adequately fund the Indian Health Service.[2] The lack of federal coverage and fear of non-Indian providers has resulted in a health disparity that is greater between the American Indian and the general population than any other race or ethnicity.

Reliance on native traditional healers has continued for many reservation-based Indian populations. Although most spiritual healing ceremonies were considered unlawful in the United States until the American Indian Religious Freedom Act of 1978, the use of such practices continued in secret and on a limited basis. As diseases occurred that were new to the aboriginal people, the need to reach out to Western medicine increased. Immunizations were given in hopes of reducing infectious diseases. Although the concept of putting sickness in to keep sickness out was very foreign, the desire to reduce the number of people dying slowly overcame the fear. Gradually, other services were used and expanded. It remains today that with some tribal groups, there are diseases or ailments that are for "white doctors" and some for traditional healers. Individuals rarely see a conflict in using both systems. Often a person will seek a traditional healer and a physician for the same complaint, but for different aspects of the condition.

Most American Indian tribes believe that illness is a result of an imbalance in the 4 cardinal aspects of a person: mind, body, heart/emotion, and spirit. Because Western medicine predominantly focuses on the physical condition, traditional healers strive to bring the other elements into balance. It is not unusual for an individual to feel that it is important to bring the balance back into place before seeking the physical remedy, believing that the condition will only return if balance is not achieved. The method of restoring balance is unique to each tribe or tribal group.

As more and more American Indians were removed from reservations and placed in urban settings as a policy of assimilation, most lost contact with their traditions or the ability to live in accordance with them. Unfortunately, the loss of the traditional system was not quickly or easily replaced with the adoption of an urban non-Indian system. Indian people often feel not only the loss of a health provider but of that which keeps them in balance. While approximately 60% of the Indian population now live off reservations, for many the urban experience is extremely trying and establishes a mobility pattern of trying to go home to connect with family and culture and then back to the city for work. The disjointedness that results increases the challenges of the family and the health system in establishing consistent quality care.

Communication patterns differ among many tribes and greatly influence the ability or willingness to participate in a prescribed treatment. In many tribal belief systems, words are very powerful, and action follows words, meaning that words affect future events. Conversely, in standard English, words are used to describe action but have little influence on events. This results in the need for a provider to carefully phrase the conversation in the positive (eg, "By eating a healthy diet, your baby will be strong." rather than "If you don't take vitamins, your baby may be sick."). When death or illness must be discussed, the use of third person is helpful ("How do you think a woman would want her baby cared for if he or she were born with spina bifida?"). It is important to realize that there is no greater value in Indian culture than that of a newborn. It represents the future of a people who historically have struggled to ensure a continuance.

Regardless of the culture or the cultural beliefs, all women desire an uncomplicated birth of a healthy baby at the conclusion of a pregnancy. The challenge for health professionals is working transculturally to develop an understanding of the woman's perceptions of what will lead to a safe passage. A lack of adherence to treatment or poor compliance is often misinterpreted as not willing to do what is necessary for a healthy baby when it may simply reflect the woman's conviction of some other need for her infant. Still it is a misconception to think that the practices and beliefs of American Indians/Alaskan Natives can be lumped into one group. Each tribe among the more than 500 federally recognized tribes has its own traditions; some groups may be similar, but great differences may occur between distinct tribes such as the Lakota and Navajo. For example, the lifestyles associated with hunter/gatherers versus dwellers contribute to different customs, including those related to childbirth. This chapter will present information on 2 separate groups: the Crow, representing the Northern Plains, and a combination of Northern Ute, Shoshone, and Paiute as Great Basin tribes. Even among these groups, practices may differ among families or clans; thus to the degree generalities can be made, common themes of perinatal health care will be presented.

The Crow Tribe

Pregnancy/Prenatal Care

While prenatal care is seen as important, the need for early prenatal care is not seen as critical. Pregnancy is considered a healthy state not requiring a physician or medical provider. Women will seek care to prepare for the delivery as the pregnancy continues. The role of clan uncle is very important during the prenatal period. Clan uncles are patrilineal clan members who are very protective of the pregnant woman.[3] The clan uncle is asked to pray for the health of the child and for an easy delivery. He will be available to the woman throughout her pregnancy to help with prayers and support.

In an attempt to minimize disappointment if something happens during pregnancy and the baby dies, a crow mother does not usually prepare in advance for the infant. The husband and the grandparents are responsible for getting the necessary things ready after the baby is born. Many of the items needed are available through an extended family network. Using hand-me-down clothes is seen as a positive option and helps keep sickness away. For other items, baby showers are given after the baby is born.

Eating clay is not an unusual practice, although not done routinely by all women.[3] The ingestion of small bits of clay reduces heartburn and food cravings. The clay used is a specific type of white clay found along riverbeds. There are no specific foods that need to be avoided during pregnancy. Crow women still practice the use of sweat baths to assist in general health and to promote an easier labor. The baths are used at least weekly throughout the pregnancy. A sweat lodge is used in which hot rocks are placed in the center of a small covered hut and water poured over them to create steam.

Labor and Delivery

Most Crow women are now comfortable with delivering in a hospital setting with assistance from health care professionals. In contrast, the role of men has not changed as much. Crow men traditionally do not participate in the labor and delivery. However, it is becoming more common for men to be present during labor and, occasionally, during delivery if they are comfortable with that expanded role. The pregnant woman's mother is the most common person to accompany the woman during labor and delivery.

Peyote is often given to the woman by the clan uncle as her labor begins. The practice of using peyote during labor is described as a religious part of the Native American Church and is intended to make the birth process safer and the baby healthier.[3] In hospitals serving women from Indian communities known to follow the practices of the Native American Church, it is common to ask about peyote use prior to giving routine labor medications. Peyote is used again several months following the birth of a healthy child to give thanks.

Postpartum and Newborn Care

Traditional practices concerning the care of the umbilical cord still exist. The cord is saved when it falls off and put in a small leather square. It is beaded and worn on the girl's ceremonial dress or the boy's beaded belt. The wearing of the cord is thought to ensure the health of the child. Another old custom involves placing the cord on an anthill to prevent "jitteriness" in the baby.[3]

Anglican names are now given to babies at the time of birth. If a woman chooses to name her child in the traditional Crow way, a name is given 4 days after the birth. Some families still choose to use traditional naming ceremonies, but they are losing their significance.

Learning to care for the newborn is taught by the grandmother, who usually lives in the same house or within close proximity. She is an integral part of the pregnancy, delivery, and care of the child. The grandmother may raise the first child to show the mother what needs to be done. The role of the grandmother continues, resulting in a multigenerational family unit.

Family Planning

While breastfeeding at one time provided a means of birth control, it is becoming less popular due to the demands on the contemporary woman. Thus other means of birth control are now being sought.

Perinatal Health Care Issues of Crow Women: Key Highlights

Prenatal Care
- Pregnancy is considered a healthy state not requiring the immediate attention of a medical provider.

Pregnancy Diet
- Eating clay is not an unusual practice although not done by all women.

Labor and Delivery
- The pregnant woman's mother is the most common support person during labor and birth.
- Peyote is often given to the woman by the clan uncle as her labor begins.

Neonatal Care
- The umbilical cord is saved when it falls off and is worn by the child to ensure his or her health.
- Newborn care is taught by the grandmother.

Breastfeeding/Breast Care
- Breastfeeding is no longer a priority among Crow women.

Ute, Paiute, and Shoshone Tribes

Pregnancy/Prenatal Care

While prenatal care is valued, it is not often that a woman will seek care in the first trimester because it is viewed as risking a miscarriage or compromising the baby's health to talk about it during the first trimester. Thus it is not announced to the community until after the third month to ensure that the mother stays calm and the baby healthy.

Diagnostic testing is viewed as invading the baby and his or her unique environment. Many believe that it is not good to expose the fetus to "currents" such as ultrasound. The fetus is safe within his or her natural habitat and that habitat should be protected.

Fathers usually do not go to doctors' appointments with the pregnant mother. Sisters, aunts, or her mother accompany her. Most major decisions will be made by the grandmothers or after talking with them.

Although many of the traditions regarding food are no longer observed, a few remain. Indian women have instinctively recognized certain foods as good for the baby and identified others as harmful. Fish, for example, continues to be thought a good dietary source of protein and essential oils during pregnancy. A pregnant woman following traditional practices does not eat wild game, cold foods or drink, or sweet foods such as gum or candy. The ban on sweet foods may be an adaptation to the exceedingly high rate of diabetes among this population and its potential risk to the baby.

Traditional beliefs related to pregnancy still exist and several are followed to this day. Even when certain practices are not believed to be harmful to the baby, an attitude of "better safe than sorry" seems to persist. For example, funerals, scary movies, and bad thoughts usually are avoided by pregnant women because they may upset the mother and, thus, negatively effect the baby. Other beliefs include the following: wearing necklaces or belts may strangle the baby or cause the cord to wrap around its neck; the stomach protects the baby, and should not be touched by others; the sacred place of the baby is to be kept private and it is not good to talk about how much it moves or kicks; privacy also helps the mother remain calm; and music is beneficial to the fetus, and a mother often will sing or provide other music during pregnancy to make for a more pleasant baby once it is born.

Labor and Delivery

The role of men and women in labor and delivery is fairly traditional. Often it is only the women of the family who are present during labor and delivery. If men are in the room, they may not touch their own hair or face or that of the mother. They should also not look in the mirror until the umbilical cord falls off.

Children are not in attendance at the birth. Contemporary medicines are usually not used during labor. Taking a long hot bath or staying in a warm bath is customary. Men usually take the mother for a long "bumpy" ride before going to the hospital. While at one time home birth was a common occurrence, it is now routine to deliver in a hospital setting. Spiritual rituals or ceremonies are preferred to be done at home after the mother and baby leave the hospital.

Postpartum and Newborn Care

The woman and infant are expected to stay at home for 30 days after the birth, and company is discouraged. If people outside the family come to the home, the mother and baby will usually leave the room. Fathers, siblings, and women of the extended family are very involved with the baby; however, the women do most of the care for the new mother and her newborn. Breastfeeding is very important for women today. It is seen more as a feeding practice than a birth control method, but continues to help space children.

It is important for infants to be wrapped very tightly from the beginning, and they are often placed on cradle boards. This increases the baby's sense of well-being. While cradle boards were traditionally used for several months, up to a year, they are now usually used for only the first month. It is still common practice not to cut the baby's hair for the first year.

Umbilical cords are saved, and a variety of customs surround keeping the cord. It can be wrapped in leather and placed on the crib or cradle board, it can be put out on an anthill and left for the ants to consume, or it can be buried near the family home. If the umbilical cord is not taken care of properly, many believe that the child will always be searching for a sense of belonging. If a person were habitually restless, one would assume that their cord had not been properly cared for as an infant. It would reflect back on the mother. Placentas are not used for any ceremonial or spiritual practice and are rarely taken from the hospital.

A traditional practice that has mostly been abandoned is the avoidance of bathing the infant for the first month. There was also an old practice of not cutting a newborn's fingernails. If nails are cut, the thought was that the baby would grow up to be a thief. Circumcision is currently a voluntary practice and is solely dependent on the choice of the parents.

Naming ceremonies are frequently held when the family feels it is the right time. Both an English and Indian name are given. The Indian name usually reflects something that occurs on that day. Grandmothers are often involved in choosing or approving the name chosen for a child. It would not be appropriate to name the baby after someone who is still alive.

Around the time a child reaches his or her first birthday, a common practice involves a sudden and short exposure to very cold water. A mother may dip the naked child in a creek or roll him or her quickly in snow. This is thought to make them stronger in life.

It is common for infants and young children to sleep with their parents. It is used as a bonding time and provides a sense of security for the young child. A child as old as 4 years may still be sleeping with parents or at least falling asleep with them and perhaps being moved to his or her own bed after he or she is asleep. This is a strongly held belief with no indication that changing it would benefit either the child or the parents.

Family Planning

An elder of the Ute tribe reported that when a young woman experiences her first menstrual period, she spends that time away from her family in a lodging set aside for this purpose. This was thought to help the elders live a long time. The practice is no longer followed.

It is thought to be beneficial to have children with a 3- to 4-year separation between them. This would give the mother's body time to recuperate and allow time with the young child for bonding and teaching. Breastfeeding was seen as a way to space pregnancies. Elders also speak of the men knowing that it was not right to engage in sexual relationships with the mother while she was breastfeeding. While not followed as closely as some believe is necessary, the belief remains that children are not as healthy if they are born close together.

Older traditional women are concerned about the use of birth control pills, but it is becoming acceptable with the younger generations. The use of hormone implants or intrauterine devices (IUDs) is considered unhealthy, and very few women are comfortable with these approaches to family planning.

Death/Burial Rites

Miscarriages are dealt with in the same manner as the death of a child, regardless of the age of the fetus. The fetus/infant is named and receives the same consideration by having a community funeral and any ceremonies that might be held for an older child or adult. Mourning customs are also observed for a miscarriage as well as an infant death. The full family participates in the 1-year observance of mourning. Family members will cut their hair as a symbol of loss. Some tribal activities involve a 4-day wake soon after the funeral. The avoidance of cold food and drink is common after a miscarriage.

Perinatal Health Care Issues of Ute, Paiute, and Shoshone Women: Key Highlights

Prenatal Care

- Some believe that talking about the baby before the first trimester ends can be harmful to the baby's health.
- Sisters, aunts, or her mother accompanies the mother to prenatal visits.

Prenatal Testing

- Diagnostic testing is viewed as invasive to the baby's unique environment. This includes ultrasound and amniocentesis.

Pregnancy Diet

- A pregnant woman following traditional practices does not eat wild game, cold foods or drinks, or sweet foods such as gum or candy.

Pregnancy-Related Beliefs/Taboos

- Pregnant women should not attend funerals.
- There is a concern that wearing necklaces or belts could lead to the umbilical cord wrapping around the baby's neck.
- It is important to protect the baby's environment, and it is not good to have many people feeling the mother's stomach.

Labor and Delivery
- After labor begins, a long warm or hot bath is customary.
- While it was common to give birth at home, it is now a routine to deliver in a hospital.

Postpartum Care
- The woman and infant are expected to stay at home for 30 days after the birth.

Neonatal Care
- Cradle boards are still common during the first month to provide a sense of well-being for the infant.
- Umbilical cords are kept when they fall off.
- It is common for infants and young children to sleep with their parents.

Breastfeeding/Breast Care
- Breastfeeding is encouraged and felt to be very important.

Family Planning
- Older traditional women are concerned about the use of birth control pills; however, it is becoming acceptable with the younger generations.
- The use of hormone implants or IUDs is considered unhealthy.

Death/Burial Rites
- Miscarriages are viewed as the same as an infant death.
- Practices and periods of mourning are observed as if an older child had died.
- Avoidance of cold food and drink is common after a miscarriage.

References

1. Kauffman JA. *Reauthorization of the Indian Health Care Improvement Act, Background and Issues.* Menlo Park, CA: Henry J. Kaiser Family Foundation; 1999:8–10
2. Cox D, Langwell K, Topoleski C, Green JH. *Sources of Financing and the Level of Health Spending for Native Americans.* Menlo Park, CA: Henry J. Kaiser Family Foundation; 1999:7
3. Harding R. *Traditional Beliefs and Behaviors Affecting Childbearing Practices of Crow Indian Women* [master's thesis]. Bozeman, MT: Montana State University; 1981:58–70

Further Reading

Waxman A. Navajo childbirth in transition. *Med Anthropol.* 1990;12:187–206

Acknowledgment

Acknowledgment is made to the Utah Indian Health Advisory Board for the information on Great Basin practices.

14
Perinatal Health Care Issues of Pakistani Women

Iffath Abbasi Hoskins

The racial and ethnic composition of the population in the United States has changed significantly during recent years. Between 1990 and 2000 there was a 74% increase in the Asian population, and, according to the US census for 2000, 3.6% of the more than 281 million inhabitants in the United States were Asian.[1] This figure encompasses an increasingly diverse populace with countless cultural differences that distinguish them.[2]

Culture is a broad term encompassing collectively held ideas, concepts, beliefs, values, and goals, and can include common race, ethnicity, socioeconomic level, gender, religion, profession, sexual orientation, age, etc. According to Hofstede,[3] culture is the collective programming of the human mind, distinguishing the members of one group from those of another. Wells[4] further defines it as the shared experiences and commonalities that evolve under changing social and political environments. Regardless of its definition, individuals from similar backgrounds may take on distinctly different cultural identities; this is commonplace among young versus old and rural versus urban people. During every health care encounter, the culture of the patient, the provider, and the medical institution will affect utilization, compliance, and, eventually, the health outcomes.[2] Providers can best serve their patients by increasing their understanding and awareness of the cultures they serve and by being open-minded about those unfamiliar to them.

Cultural awareness, or a lack thereof, may help or hinder how different groups interact with one another. Such awareness must include an objective and nonjudgmental view toward beliefs, actions, practices, and lifestyles. As a case in point, a recent survey conducted by the American Social Health Association[5] found that 20% of the female participants avoid gynecologic care due to language and cultural differences; this may be due to perceived cultural discord between themselves and their providers.

More than 90% of Pakistanis are Muslim. Based on their cultural and religious beliefs, they tend to have a fatalistic attitude toward life and attribute all things that happen as the will of God. In a positive sense, this allows them to not question life but rather to accept God's will but, in a negative sense, it diminishes the need for them to be proactive and involved in their own well-being.

Fewer than 30% of Pakistani immigrants lived in a city in their native land. Less than 15% are literate, and an even smaller percentage are fluent in English. In traditional families, females are raised to be quiet, meek, and subservient to males; they are expected to help run the household and care for other family members, especially parents and other elders. Furthermore, they are often considered a burden because they have to be fed and nurtured, using up the meager family resources only to be turned over to another family at marriage, which only incurs additional costs. Thus throughout their upbringing, girls tend to be treated as second-class citizens, being given less food, less attention, and fewer amenities than their brothers and fathers. As a result, the nutritional status of Pakistani women is frequently substandard, many believing that they have no rights and should have no expectations. Most importantly, they are married off at very young ages (usually by age 13 years) and often to men far older than themselves.

In a survey of 150 random women, Fikree and Bhatti[6] discovered through confidential interviews that 34% had been abused in the past and that 15% had been abused during pregnancy; 72% of the abused women reported anxiety and/or depression. Thus domestic violence poses a serious health problem in Pakistan.

When Pakistani women immigrate to a Western nation, new conflicts often arise. They may find themselves on the lower end of the
socioeconomic spectrum and may encounter language, religious, and
cultural barriers. In addition, not only do they lose their place in a
familiar society, but they also lose the kinship and support of other
females that they used to have in their native land. Above all, they lose
the main role by which they define themselves (ie, one of providing
kinship and support to others in their families and communities,
while making their own needs subservient). They may, therefore,
exhibit a lingering combination of sadness and confusion, even
though they themselves may be relatively safe and well cared for in
their adopted land. Furthermore, once they are exposed to Western
influences, which include increased freedoms for themselves and their
children within the household and immigrant community, they still
must maintain the traditional norms of subservience and passivity.
This can be confusing to them.

Health and Illness

In Pakistan, maternal and infant mortality is high and life expectancy
is low. Overall, the estimated maternal mortality rate in Pakistan is
433 per 100,000 live births.[7] This varies between 281 for Karachi
(a highly industrialized city) to 673 in the rural and remote portions
of the country. The 3 leading, but generally preventable, causes are
hemorrhage (53%), sepsis (16%), and eclampsia (14%). Other cau-
sative factors include poor construction of houses and buildings,
leading to poor sanitation; more than 40 miles to the nearest hospital;
and grand multiparity.

Many men have more than one spouse. Others may be in homosexual relationships that are unknown to the wife. Homosexuality is
extremely shunned and hidden within Islamic societies. The wife usually has no way of knowing who her husband's partners are or were.
Additionally, she has no right to ask him. Thus she is at very high risk
of transmission of sexually transmitted diseases (STDs), having almost

no options to prevent or decrease those risks, and illnesses such as pelvic inflammatory disease are common. There is also no national program in Pakistan to address the human immunodeficiency virus (HIV) epidemic. Similar gender-related attitudes affect infertility workups as well. It is almost unheard of for a male to accept responsibility for a couple's infertility. All such interventions and treatments, as well as any blame for the problem, are considered the responsibility of the female.

Physicians in Pakistan often cover more than one area hospital while maintaining lucrative private practices that keep them quite busy. Thus those patients who cannot afford the expensive private medical care generally receive care from recently graduated, and not very experienced, doctors who work without much supervision and oversight; and these are usually the sickest patients. Many Pakistanis prefer homeopathic or alternative health care practices and may be confused by Western medicine. Thus there may be a clash between these 2 systems, and the patient may be caught between conflicting ideas.

Pregnancy/Prenatal Care

Pakistani women tend to be very young when they first become pregnant, and the demands of pregnancy and lactation may compromise their own developing bodies. In addition, they usually have many children and the strains of numerous pregnancies and breastfeeding, coupled with poor nutrition, often take a further toll on their health and well-being. Thus serious complications related to pregnancy and childbirth often ensue, resulting in high maternal and infant mortality. Of the ones who survive, many have long-term sequelae due to the fact that in rural Pakistan, pregnant women are usually cared for by lay midwives in out-of-hospital settings where skilled medical interventions, anesthesia, operative obstetrics, blood transfusions, etc, are unavailable. Once in the United States, these women will accept most screening tests and procedures without question; however, they will usually refuse any intervention that could negatively affect their pregnancy.

Abortion is almost never chosen as an option, regardless of the problems of pregnancy or deformities that are identified in the fetus. A 1997 study of the characteristics of 452 Pakistani women seeking abortion in a 3-month period showed that 8.6% were unmarried, 37% were older than 35 years, 61% had more than 5 children, and 40% were illiterate[8]; furthermore, nearly two thirds of the abortions were conducted by inadequately trained personnel (as defined by World Health Organization criteria).[9]

There are very few preventive and screening programs in Pakistan; thus immigrants to the United States usually do not seek out preventive health care services. Even during their pregnancies, their accessing of the system is usually dependent on, and subservient to, the greater perceived needs of their families. As such, they may not seek prenatal care until late in the pregnancy or only at the time of delivery. In a survey of 711 women who delivered singleton pregnancies from 1994 to 1995, Pakistani women made 9.1% fewer antenatal visits than white British women.[10]

Medical conditions such as thalassemias and other hemoglobinopathies are high, occurring in approximately 25% of the population. Beta thalassemia is one of the most common inherited single gene disorders in Pakistan. It is characterized by reduced or absent beta globin gene expression, resulting in abnormal maturation and survival of red blood cells. There are 5 common mutations among Pakistanis that result in a high likelihood of hydrops fetalis and other fetal complications. But, because of social/cultural constraints, the women rarely undergo any testing or other interventions. Moreover, identifying carrier status in the spouse is practically impossible because husbands traditionally shirk any and all responsibilities for medical outcomes of the family.

Ahmed et al[11] described a strategy for identifying and counseling carriers of recessively inherited disorders in developing countries where consanguineous marriages are common. In such communities, gene variants are trapped within extended families, so that an affected child is a marker for a group at high genetic risk. Ten large families with carriers and affected individuals were screened for hemoglobinopathies (including beta thalassemia) and were compared with 5 control families. No carrier was found among the 397 individuals tested. However, of the 591 individuals in the at-risk groups, 31% were carriers and 8% of married couples were both carriers. All carriers reportedly used the information to either avoid further pregnancies or to access prenatal diagnosis, if indicated. Model et al[12] reported that residents of Pakistani origin are now the main group at risk for beta thalassemia in the United Kingdom. The proportion of affected births remains 50% higher than would be expected, reflecting a widespread failure to deliver timely screening and counseling to carriers.

Vangen et al[13] compared 66 Pakistani women with 71 Norwegian women for antenatal outcomes and complications. They found that the Pakistani women had higher rates of gestational diabetes (crude OR = 5.0, 95% CI = 1.5–20.5), intrauterine growth retardation (crude OR = 5.0, 95% CI = 1.4–18.8), hyperemesis gravidarum (crude OR = 3.7, 95% CI = 1.1–12.2), anemia (crude OR = 10.2, 95% CI = 3.3–31.4), and congenital malformations (P = .048). The Norwegian women had higher rates of physical complaints such as pelvic pain (crude OR = 0.4, 95% CI = 0.2–0.8) and exhaustion (crude OR = 0.2, 95% CI = 0.04–0.1). Infections such as tuberculosis (TB) and hepatitis only occurred in the Pakistani women.

Many infections and communicable diseases are problematic for the Pakistani community. These include TB, hepatitis A, yellow fever, and malaria. Aziz et al[14] reviewed the cases of 53 pregnant women and found that 38% had fulminant hepatic failure, with non-A and non-B hepatitis the most common cause (occurring in 62% of the patients).

Hepatitis B occurred in 17% and hepatitis A in 4%. The case fatality rate was 15%. One of the poor prognostic factors was lack of antenatal care. Drug-resistant TB is another problem. Once in the United States, these patients will be screened and, if necessary, treated for long periods. Such prolonged treatments can be a challenge for any family, but are especially cumbersome for Pakistani women given their cultural and religious constraints.

Naim and Bhutto[15] studied 150 healthy pregnant Pakistanis regarding patterns of sexual activity during pregnancy. Although attitudes were mixed, they found a tilt toward believing that coitus should be avoided during the third trimester of pregnancy.

Pakistani women readily eat nutritious foods, including meats, vegetables, and dairy products. However, they have many religious constraints, which include eating only kosher meats and poultry that have been slaughtered in a specific way and avoiding pork and shellfish. They also try to avoid lard or other pork products that are sometimes used as food additives. Medications that are derived from pigs, such as vitamins and insulin, may be exempt from these dietary restrictions.

Vitamin D deficiency is widespread among Pakistani women. It may cause damage to the maternal pelvis and, thus, may be a risk factor for cephalopelvic disproportion (CPD). Brunvand et al[16] compared vitamin D blood levels between 37 nulliparas who had cesarean sections for CPD with 80 nulliparas with uncomplicated vaginal deliveries. They found that mothers with obstructed labors were shorter (150 vs 155 cm, $P = .001$) and lighter (58 kg vs 60.5 kg, $P = .005$); 71% of all the patients had low or low to normal vitamin D values (<30 mmol/L). However, vitamin D deficiency occurred equally in the 2 groups (20 out of 37 obstructed labor patients and 63 out of 80 controls). They concluded that, in spite of nutritional (and dietary) preferences in Pakistan, vitamin D deficiency did not adversely affect obstetric outcomes.

In a different study, Brunvand et al[17] reviewed fetal growth outcomes in 30 vitamin D–deficient pregnant mothers. Although all of the women had uncomplicated pregnancies and deliveries, nearly all of them (96.7%) had decreased vitamin D blood levels (<30 mmol/L), and there was a correlation between the low vitamin D levels and low crown-heel lengths of the infants. These investigators also reported that only 33% of the women who received free vitamin D actually ingested it. Furthermore, 56% of the women given the free vitamins still had deficient vitamin D levels, as did 76% of the controls who did not receive free vitamins. Thus it was shown that just giving free vitamins without patient education is of questionable value.

Compliance regarding nutrition, rest, medications, etc, during pregnancy is often dictated by the tendency for Pakistani women to put the needs of their husbands and children above their own. Frequently, they live in the homes of their husbands' parents, and their mothers-in-law may be extremely demanding and unkind, often disregarding the pregnant woman's special needs, considering it their inherent right to inflict suffering on their daughters-in-law because they suffered themselves at the hands of their own mothers-in-law.

Pakistani husbands, fathers, or brothers are usually not involved in any part of the pregnancy, childbirth, or postpartum period. It is also rare for women to receive medical care from males. It may, thus, be distressing, and a potential source of conflict within their households, when they cannot always choose the gender of their health care providers in the United States. In general, they are usually too subdued to question or disagree with a proposed regimen and will rarely admit to having an unsupportive or abusing spouse.

Labor and Delivery
In Pakistan, female relatives are the main source of support before, during, and after a woman gives birth. Once in the United States, it is usually left to the woman alone to handle all of the health care issues of her pregnancy as well as those of her family.

Pakistani women have a unique way of responding to personal and physical discomfort. It can vary from stoicism (where they try to avoid public displays of emotions and feelings) to being unrestrained in showing their feelings, but not voicing any feelings. Thus it is not uncommon to see a laboring woman grimacing as if in intense physical pain and with tears streaming down her face, but refusing to complain or describe her pain. Vangen et al[18] compared 67 Pakistani women to 70 Norwegian women regarding their use of analgesics during labor. They found that 30% of the Pakistani women did not receive labor analgesia compared with 9% of Norwegian women. When adjusted for age, parity, and duration of labor, Pakistani origin was the only significant predictor for no labor analgesia.

Vangen et al[13] also state that a mother's ethnicity is associated with her baby's birth weight and risk of perinatal mortality. They reviewed data for more than 808,000 births in Norway from 1980 to 1995. Of these, 6,854 were Pakistani, and their mean birth weights were low (3,244 g) versus those reported for the Norwegians (3530 g). Perinatal mortality was highest among Pakistanis (14.9/1,000) versus 9.5 per 1,000 for Norwegians.

Postpartum and Newborn Care

In the Pakistani culture, family and friends provide extensive support after childbirth. The new mother rarely has to care for the newborn. Such duties are usually taken over by the elder (more experienced) women in the family. If there is no female family member available, other "elder" females in the community (even though they are not related) take over these duties. In the United States, she must perform all self-care and baby care without the customary help. Thus she may feel ambivalent about her recovery, which may add to her emotional stress. The husband is almost never involved except as an observer.

The new mother is discouraged from bathing due to the belief that washing the hair creates a cold sensation for the body and adversely affects her healing and recovery. Additionally, she is taught to avoid cleaning her breasts and nipples for the same reasons. This clearly affects her personal hygiene. Therefore, much attention must be focused on teaching her basic bathing and other hygiene practices. New mothers are expected to not leave their homes. This is for numerous reasons, including a superstition that there may be "evil spirits" or a "black magic" spell that can affect the mother and her newborn and a belief that exposure to the "cool" outside atmosphere might interfere with her recovery and healing process.

The new mother is encouraged to choose a "nutritious" diet that would help her recovery while nourishing her newborn. These include foods thought to target the baby's central nervous system, and include walnuts, pecans, almonds, etc. Fresh fruits and vegetables are also favored, legumes are thought to have little nutritious value, and cold products are avoided. The new mother prefers that the room temperature and her environment remain "hot" because warming is thought to result in accelerating her recovery process. Most babies are breastfed for up to 1 to 2 years of life. However, when the mother's nutrition is substandard, the long-term effects can be detrimental to both mother and baby.

When a woman bleeds vaginally, she is considered to be unclean and cannot engage in sexual intercourse or participate in religious activities (such as prayers). Once the bleeding (postpartal or menstrual) stops, she must bathe and shave her underarms and pubic hair to cleanse herself. Only then can she pray or have relations with her husband.

There are many customs and ceremonies involving newborn care. Many of these are harmless. For instance, the baby is named within 72 hours of birth in a ceremony involving the father or grandfather reciting the *Aazan* (a prayer) in the baby's ear. Male babies are preferred, especially as firstborns, and all are circumcised. The mother (or other female family member) must be taught appropriate care of the surgical site as well as the umbilical cord. By the third day, the baby's head is shaved in a special ceremony because the hair that the baby had within the mother's womb is considered especially vulnerable to "black magic." This hair, once removed, is not discarded as trash. Rather, it is either buried under a tree or thrown into a river as protection from evil spirits. Additionally, all newborns are made to wear a thick black string either around the neck or wrist. Again, this is meant to ward off evil spells and spirits.

While 95% of all new mothers initiate breastfeeding, only 16% exclusively breastfeed by 3 months, and only 56% of mothers are still breastfeeding their babies at all by 24 months.[19] Ojha[20] sampled 300 women aged 20 to 35 years in India to assess religious differences in childbirth and childrearing practices. Muslim women had similarly high rates of breastfeeding as their Hindu and Christian counterparts, but they had the lowest rates of being loving toward and protective of their children. The authors suggested that this may be due to their passive and fatalistic approaches to life.

Family Planning

Male contraceptives (eg, condoms) are almost never used in Pakistan. In rural communities, women either do not use contraceptives or do so without the knowledge or permission of their husbands; thus any spacing of children tends to be unplanned or coincides with the periods of pregnancy and lactation. Abortion is generally not considered an option. Young (30 years of age or younger), urban, literate Pakistani women of high economic status whose mothers-in-law reported discussing family planning with them and who received family planning information from health care workers were 2 to 3 times more likely to use contraceptives than other women.[21]

Death/Burial Rites

Death and illness are accepted in a fatalistic manner as being the will of God. However, because most families are encouraged to be joyous during the childbirth period, if there is a death or other mishap in the family, the new mother and child are discouraged from being present in the areas where the mourning occurs because any sadness is thought to attract bad or dangerous vibes that could hurt them or even result in death.

Every Pakistani Woman Is Unique

Understanding cultural issues will assist the provider in drawing out the Pakistani woman so that she may become more involved in her own care. Many immigrants are homesick, not only for their own culture but also for the support systems they left behind. Their illiteracy and stoicism combine to create an impression of cooperation and passivity. This must be acknowledged and addressed to provide the woman with appropriate and accurate medical care for her and her baby.

Perinatal Health Care Issues of Pakistani Women: Key Highlights

Demographic/Psychosocial/Spiritual Characteristics

- More than 90% of Pakistanis are Muslim.
- Fewer than 30% of Pakistani immigrants lived in a city in their native land.
- Fewer than 15% are literate, and an even smaller percentage are fluent in English.
- Medical conditions such as thalassemias and other hemoglobinopathies are high, occurring in approximately 25% of the population.
- The estimated maternal mortality rate in Pakistan is 433 per 100,000 live births.
- In traditional families, females are raised to be quiet, meek, and subservient to males.
- Based on their cultural and religious beliefs, they tend to have a fatalistic attitude to life and attribute all things that happen as the will of God.

Prenatal Care

- Compliance regarding nutrition, rest, medications, etc, during pregnancy is often dictated by the tendency for Pakistani women to put the needs of their husbands and children above their own; thus they may not seek prenatal care until late in the pregnancy or only at the time of delivery.
- Pakistani women will usually accept prenatal tests or procedures as long as an intervention will not negatively affect their pregnancy.
- In rural Pakistan, pregnant women are usually cared for by lay midwives in out-of-hospital settings, where skilled medical interventions, anesthesia, operative obstetrics, blood transfusions, etc, are unavailable.

Pregnancy Diet

- Although they readily eat nutritious foods, including meats, vegetables, and dairy products, vitamin D deficiency is widespread among Pakistani women.

Pregnancy-Related Beliefs/Taboos

- The newborn's hair is considered especially vulnerable to "black magic." It is removed within 3 days and either buried under a tree or thrown into a river as protection from evil spirits.
- All newborns are made to wear a thick black string either around the neck or wrist. Again, this is meant to ward off evil spells and spirits.

Labor and Delivery

- Female relatives are the main source of support for the Pakistani woman during labor.
- The response of Pakistani women to pain in labor can vary from stoicism to an unrestrained display of discomfort, while not voicing their feelings.
- In Pakistan, analgesia during labor is not the norm.

Postpartum Diet

- The new mother's diet includes foods thought to target the baby's central nervous system (eg, walnuts, pecans, almonds, etc).
- Fresh fruits and vegetables are favored; legumes are not considered nutritious.
- Cold products are avoided.

Postpartum Care

- In Pakistan, family and friends provide extensive support after childbirth; the new mother rarely has to care for the newborn; in the United States, she must do all self-care and tend to the baby without the customary help.
- The new mother is discouraged from bathing due to the belief that washing the hair creates a cold sensation for the body and adversely affects her healing and recovery.
- The room temperature and environment should remain "hot" because warming is thought to result in accelerating the woman's recovery process.
- The Pakistani woman cannot engage in sexual intercourse or participate in any religious activity until the postpartal bleeding stops; then, she must bathe and shave her underarms and pubic hair before resuming prayer or relations with her husband.

Neonatal Care

- Most Pakistani babies are breastfed for up to 1 to 2 years of life.
- The baby is named within 72 hours of birth in a ceremony involving the father or grandfather reciting the *Aazan* (a prayer) in the baby's ear.
- Male babies are preferred, especially as firstborns.
- By the third day, the baby's head is shaved in a special ceremony.
- All males are circumcised in Pakistan.

Breastfeeding/Breast Care

- The initiation of breastfeeding is almost universal among Pakistani women, but supplemental feeding is commonly added within the first 3 months.
- The new mother is discouraged from cleaning her breasts and nipples immediately after giving birth.

Pregnancy Termination/Miscarriage

- Elective abortion is usually not an acceptable option for an undesired pregnancy.

Family Planning

- Male contraceptives (eg, condoms) are almost never used.
- In rural communities, women generally do not use contraceptives or do so without the knowledge or permission of their husbands; thus any spacing of children is unplanned or coincides with the periods of pregnancy and lactation.

Death/Burial Rites

- Death is accepted in a fatalistic manner as being the will of God.
- A new mother and child avoid being around any mourning because sadness is thought to attract bad or dangerous vibes that could hurt them or even result in death.

References

1. US Bureau of the Census. *Statistical Abstract of the US* Washington, DC: US Bureau of the Census; 2000. Available at: http://www.census.gov/ population/www/cen2000/phc-tl. Accessed February 1, 2003
2. ACOG committee opinion. *Cultural competency in health care.* Number 201, March 1998. Committee on Health Care for Underserved Women. American College of Obstetricians and Gynecologists. *Int J Gynaecol Obstet.* 1998;62:96–99
3. Hofstede G. *Cultures and Organizations, Softwares of the Mind. Intercultural Cooperation and Its Importance for Survival.* New York, NY: McGraw-Hill; 1997

4. Wells MI. Beyond cultural competence: a model for individual and institutional cultural development. *J Community Health Nurs.* 2000;17:189–199

5. American Social Health Association. *Reasons Why Women Avoid Seeking Gynecologic Healthcare.* Available at: http://www.ashastd.org/news/gynsurvey.html. Accessed April 15, 2003

6. Fikree FF, Bhatti LI. Domestic violence and health of Pakistani women. *Int J Gynaecol Obstet.* 1999;65:195–201

7. Berthoud R. Teenage births to ethnic minority women. *Popul Trends.* 2001;(104):12–17

8. Fikree FF, Midhef F, Sadruddin S, Berendes HW. Maternal mortality in difficult Pakistani sites: ratios, clinical causes and determinants. *Acta Obstet Gynecol Scand.* 1997;76:637–645

9. Rehan N, Inayatullah A, Chaudhary I. Characteristics of Pakistani women seeking abortion clinics. *J Womens Health Gend Based Med.* 2001;10:805–810

10. Petrous M, Kupek E, Vanuse S, Maresh M. Clinical, provider and sociodemographic determinants of the number of antenatal visits in England & Wales. *Soc Sci Med.* 2001;52:1123–1134

11. Ahmed S, Saleem M, Model B, Petrou M. Screening extended families for genetic hemoglobin disorders in Pakistan. *N Engl J Med.* 2002;347:1200–1202

12. Model B, Khan M, Darlison M, et al. A national register for surveillance of inherited disorders: beta thalassemia in the UK *Bull World Health Org.* 2001;79:1006–1013

13. Vangen S, Stoltenberg C, Stray-Pederson B. Complaints and complications in pregnancy: a study of ethnic Norwegian and ethnic Pakistani women in Oslo. *Ethn Health.* 1999;4:19–28.

14. Aziz AB, Hamid S, Iqbal S, Islam W, Karim SA. Prevalence and severity of viral hepatitis in Pakistani pregnant women: a five year hospital based study. *J Pak Med Assoc.* 1997;47:198–201

15. Naim M, Bhutto E. Sexuality during pregnancies in Pakistani women. *J Pak Med Assoc.* 2000;50:38–44

16. Brunvand L, Shah SS, Bergstrom S, Haug E. Vitamin D deficiency in pregnancy is not associated with obstructed labour. A study among Pakistani women in Karachi. *Acta Obstet Gynecol Scand.* 1998;77:303–306

17. Brunvand L, Quigstad E, Urdal P, Haug E. Vitamin D deficiency and fetal growth. *Earth Hum Dev.* 1996;45:27–33

18. Vangen S, Stoltenberg C, Schi B. Ethnicity and use of obstetrical analgesia: do Pakistani women receive inadequate pain relief in labour? *Ethn Health.* 1996;1:161–167

19. Milking profits in Pakistan. *Multinational Monitor.* 2000;21. Available at: http://multinationalmonitor.org/mm2000/00september/front1.html. Accessed April 15, 2003

20. Ojha PM. Religion-cultural variation in childbearing practices. *Psychol Stud (Mysore).* 1992;37:65–72

21. Fikree FF, Khan A, Kadir AM, Sajan F, Rahbar MH. What influences contraceptive use among young women in urban squatter settlements of Karachi? *Int Fam Planning Perspect.* 2001;27:130–136

15
Perinatal Health Care Issues
of Seventh-Day Adventist Women

Karen K. House

Seventh-Day Adventists, also known as Adventists, are Christians. Many of the Church's founding fathers had been part of a movement in the United States during the 1830s and 1840s, believing that Jesus Christ's second coming was to occur in October 1844. When this event did not materialize, many were disappointed and left the movement; others restudied the scriptures and decided that they had misinterpreted them. Their new revelation, that Christ's second coming was some time in the future, spurred some of these believers into forming the Seventh-Day Adventist Church in 1863.

"The mission of the Adventist Church is to proclaim to all peoples the everlasting gospel in the context of the three angel's messages of Revelation 14:6–12, leading them to accept Jesus as personal Savior and to unite with His church, and nurturing them in preparation for His soon return."[1] The name *Seventh-Day Adventist* is derived from the belief that Jesus Christ is coming again (advent) and that the Biblical Sabbath is the seventh day of the week, Saturday.[1] Accordingly, the Sabbath begins Friday evening at sundown and ends Saturday evening at sundown. No work is to be done on this day of rest and worship.

Adventists believe that they will achieve their mission by preaching the gospel, educating minds and characters, healing sickness, and preserving health.[1] Since the formation of the Adventist Church, they have held true to their mission. Church membership in 1999 was nearly 11 million and was represented in 204 countries worldwide, where they provided the following services[2]:

- Education Programs
  - Total schools — 5,846
  - Tertiary institutions — 95
  - Worker training institutions — 38
  - Secondary schools — 1,115
  - Primary schools — 4,598

- Health Care Ministries
  - Hospitals and sanitariums — 166
  - Nursing homes and retirement centers — 117
  - Clinics and dispensaries — 371
  - Orphanages and children's homes — 30
  - Airplanes and medical launches — 12
  - Outpatient visits — 9.7 million

Health and Illness

Adventists believe that the human body is the temple of God. A well-accepted tenet is the following: "Along with adequate exercise and rest, we are to adopt the most healthful diet possible and abstain from the unclean foods identified in the Scriptures. Since alcoholic beverages, tobacco, and the irresponsible use of drugs and narcotics are harmful to our bodies, we are to abstain from them as well. Instead, we are to engage in whatever brings our thoughts and bodies into the discipline of Christ, who desires our wholesomeness, joy, and goodness."[3]

Many Adventists choose not to eat meat, and it is generally not served at official Adventist places or functions. However, if an Adventist does eat meat, it should be clean. Unclean foods noted in the Bible are meats from animals that do not chew cud and have cloven hoofs, any fish that does not have fins and scales, or birds that are carnivorous, such as the eagle or raven.[4] (See Box 15-1.)

Box 15-1
Adventist Food Preferences

In the Adventist vegetarian diet, protein is frequently obtained through a textured vegetable protein (wheat gluten, soy protein concentrate) product manufactured by Worthington Foods and Loma Linda Foods. The textured vegetable protein is made into substitute meat products flavored to taste like chicken, beef, or fish. These products can be fried, used like ground beef, baked, and/or broiled.

Seventh-Day Adventist health care workers strive toward preserving and restoring humans to wholeness. Rarely has the church interfered with societal practices in its worldwide church family. However, the church did make an official statement that female genital mutilation is harmful and is not justifiable as a religious practice.[5]

Pregnancy/Prenatal Care

There are no specific pregnancy, labor, birth, postpartum, or newborn care policies that Adventists must follow. Because many Adventists are vegetarians, knowing which type of vegetarian they are will help ensure that the recommended nutritional requirements are being met. If, for example, an Adventist is a lacto-ovo vegetarian (eating grains, fruits, vegetables, legumes, nuts, seeds, eggs, and dairy products), then her nutritional needs during pregnancy can be met easily.[6,7] If she is vegan vegetarian (eating grains, vegetables, fruits, seeds and nuts, legumes, but no animal products), then extra vitamin B_{12} and D supplements are recommended.[6,7]

Labor and Delivery/Postpartum and Newborn Care

Adventists observe no special traditions during childbirth or the postpartum period. In caring for their newborns, they choose from the full spectrum of options that are available to any parents within the United States.

Family Planning

The married Christian couple will need to consider religious, medical, social, and political implications when choosing a birth control method. The Adventists do consider the following birth control methods to be morally acceptable: any barrier method, spermicides, intrauterine devices (IUDs), sterilization, and hormonal methods.[8] Abortions for birth control purposes are not morally acceptable; they are deemed necessary only when used to save the life of the mother, if there is a serious genetic defect, or if the pregnancy resulted from incest and/or rape.[9] The official position on sex outside of marriage is that it is harmful and immoral.[8]

Bioethical Dilemmas

Modern Adventists face controversial life decisions similar to those confronting women and families of most religions (eg, whether to engage in premarital sex and whether to abort an unwanted pregnancy). Adventist preachers and pastors teach that waiting until marriage for sex is God's plan to live a happier healthier life, and the Church does not condone abortion for birth control. However, many Adventist women do engage in premarital sex and do use birth control. Those who become pregnant out of wedlock either opt for marriage or abortion, or choose to be single mothers. It is not necessary to confess one's transgressions to a pastor/preacher; thus the Church never needs to find out if someone is not following all of its guidelines. For most practicing Adventists, the practice "don't ask, don't tell" shields them from the Church becoming involved in their personal decisions.

There are always ethical choices to be made if there is a pregnancy that is known to be genetically or structurally defective. Because it is not against church policy to abort a pregnancy with a genetic defect, Adventist women can then make this decision a personal one with support given from family, friends, and their pastor.

Death/Burial Rites

When there is a death, Adventists do not have any special rites that they perform on the deceased. It is believed that death is an unconscious state, like sleeping, and at the Second Coming of Jesus Christ, the dead will be resurrected.[10]

A pastor is often called to a deathbed to pray for the dying person. This prayer is usually a prayer of hope, reminding the dying one that God loves him or her and that he or she will be resurrected when Jesus Christ returns. It is also a time to give courage to the family members that God is there grieving with them. But, there is hope of His second coming, when the dead will be resurrected and death and suffering will cease.

Perinatal Health Care Issues of Seventh-Day Adventist Women: Key Highlights

Demographic/Psychosocial/Spiritual Characteristics

- Church membership in 1999 was nearly 11 million and was represented in 204 countries worldwide.
- Adventists believe that they will achieve their mission by preaching the gospel, educating minds and characters, healing sickness, and preserving health.
- Baptism, the complete immersion in water, is the rite of passage into the Adventist church. This is typically done in the early teen years and any time for adult converts.
- Prayer is a direct communication with God.
- Sabbath begins sundown Friday evening and ends sundown Saturday evening. This is a day of worship, rest, and good works.
- Taking care of the body is taking care of the temple of God. Smoking, drinking, and recreational drugs are not condoned. Eating healthfully and getting enough rest and exercise are essential in taking care of this temple.

Pregnancy Diet

- Vegans (eat no animal products) need dietary supplements of 2.0 μg of vitamin B_{12} and 10 μg of vitamin D if sun exposure is limited.

Family Planning

- Barrier methods, IUDs, spermicides, sterilization, and hormones are acceptable as birth control methods; abortion as a contraceptive is not morally acceptable.

Pregnancy Termination/Miscarriage

- Pregnancy termination is deemed necessary only when used to save the life of the mother, if there is a serious genetic defect, or if the pregnancy resulted from incest and/or rape.

Bioethical Dilemmas

- Premarital sex and abortion for contraceptive purposes are not condoned practices.
- Adventists do not have to confess transgressions to their pastors.
- For structurally or genetically defective pregnancies, abortion is an option.

Death/Burial Rites

- Death is an unconscious state much like sleeping. Adventists believe that the dead will be resurrected at Jesus Christ's Second Coming.
- Most Adventists choose burial rather than cremation.

References

1. Seventh-Day Adventist Church. *Our Name and Mission.* Available at: http://www.adventist.org/name-mission/. Accessed February 1, 2003
2. Seventh-Day Adventist Church. *Facts and Figures.* Available at: http://www.adventist.org/worldchurch/factsa-ndfigures.html. Accessed February 1, 2003
3. Seventh-Day Adventist Church. *Fundamental Beliefs. #21: Christian Behavior.* Available at: http://www.adventist.org/beliefs/index.html. Accessed February 1, 2003
4. Deuteronomy.14:3–21 (KJV)
5. Seventh-Day Adventist Church. *Official Statements—Seventh-Day Adventist Statement of Consensus Concerning Female Genital Mutilation.* Available at: http://www.adventist.org/beliefs/main_stat47.html. Accessed February 1, 2003
6. American Dietetic Association. Vegetarian diets—position of ADA. *J Am Diet Assoc.* 1997;97:1317–1321. Available at: http://www.eatright.org/adap1197.html. Accessed February 1, 2003
7. American College of Obstetricians and Gynecologists. *Nutrition During Pregnancy.* Available at: http://www.medem.com/medlb/article. Accessed February 1, 2003
8. Seventh-Day Adventist Church. *Official Statements—Birth Control: A Seventh-Day Adventist Statement of Consensus.* Available at: http://www.adventist.org/beliefs/main_stat44.html. Accessed February 1, 2003
9. Seventh-Day Adventist Church. *About Adventists: Abortion.* Available at: http://www.adventist.org/beliefs/main_guide1.html. Accessed February 1, 2003
10. Seventh-Day Adventist Church. *Fundamental Beliefs. #25. Death and Resurrection.* Available at: http://www.adventist.org/beliefs/index.html. Accessed February 1, 2003

Index

A

Abortion. *See also* Pregnancy termination/
   miscarriage
   for African American women, 18
   for Cambodian women, 53
   for Chinese women, 68, 74
   for Cuban women, 108
   for Hmong women, 123
   for Jamaican women, 147
   for Japanese women, 167
   for Jewish women, 201–202
   medical ethics and, xlvii
   for Mexican women, 229
   Mormon Church on, 248, 251–252
   for Pakistani women, 275, 281
   for Seventh-Day Adventist
      women, 292
Acquired immunodeficiency syndrome
   (AIDS)
   in African Americans, 6
   in Amish, 38
   in Cambodians, 50
   in Cubans, 87, 99
   in Jamaican, 140–141
Adoption, Mormon Church on, 248
African American women
   abortion in, 18
   acquired immunodeficiency syndrome
      in, 6

alcohol use in, 6–7
bioethical dilemmas for, 18–21, 27
birth control of, 17–18
breastfeeding/breast care of, 15–16, 26
death/burial rites for, 21–23, 27
demographic characteristics of, 2,
   23–24
dietary habits of, 9–11, 25
family involvement of, 26
family planning by, 17–18, 26
geographic dispersal of, 2
health and illness of, 3–7
human immunodeficiency virus in, 6
infant mortality rates of, 8
labor and delivery of, 25
maternal mortality rate of, 7–8
miscarriage of, 27
neonatal care of, 26
nicknaming of, 15
postpartum care of, 25
pregnancy-related beliefs/taboos of, 25
prenatal care and testing of, 24
preterm birth for, xv
psychosocial characteristics of, 23–24
religious beliefs and practices of, 2,
   4–5, 26–27
self-diagnosis of, 5–6
sexually transmitted diseases of, 6
socioeconomics status of, 3